W9-CXQ-020

A WELLNESS GUIDE©

SUPREME PROPERTIES

OF

HOODIA GORDONII

Stephen Holt M.D.

**PART OF A NEW WEIGHT CONTROL REVOLUTION
IN THE COMBAT AGAINST
THE METABOLIC SYNDROME X (Y and Z...)**

www.wellnesspublishing.com

SUPREME PROPERTIES OF Hoodia GORDONII by Stephen Holt, MD
A Wellness Guide ©, Wellness Publishing, Inc.
www.wellnesspublishing.com

Book cover design: Brian Matula
Book layout: Jonathan Gullery
Editorial Assistance: Brian Matula

Manufactured in the United States
Library of Congress Cataloging-in-Publication Data.
Holt, Stephen, 1950 -

"SUPREME PROPERTIES OF HOODIA GORDONII"

ISBN: 0-9747198-0-3

Key Words: 1. Hoodia, 2. Hoodia gordonii, 3. Appetite, 4. Weight loss, 5. Obesity, 6. The metabolic Syndrome, 7. Syndrome X, 8. Alternative medicine, 9. Dietary supplements, 10. Weight control, 11. Calorie control, 12. Diet, 13. Nutrition, 14. Insulin resistance, 15. Asclepiadaceae, 16. San, 17. South Africa, 18. San bushmen, 19. Hoodia species, 20. Trichocaulon, 21. Cactus, 22.Succulent plant, 23. Diabetes mellitus, 24. Nutrition

ACKNOWLEDGEMENT

This book is a synthesis of current information on the use of Hoodia gordonii as a potential weight loss supplement, drug, or food additive. The author has searched folklore literature, scientific literature, and legal documents that are in the public realm, in order to present an overview of the biological effects of Hoodia gordonii on humans. Extracts of Hoodia gordonii are being subject to drug development pathways and it seems likely that not all scientific information, about the use of Hoodia gordonii in humans, has been completely disclosed. There has been frenetic interest in the media about the ability of Hoodia gordonii to suppress appetite and assist with weight control. I acknowledge all sources of information and much of the work reported in this book has been generated by many scientists. I have tried, where possible, to credit all sources of information. If I have failed in this regard, I apologize.

I stress that this book is not an attempt to offer a further "false promise" to many desperate people who are overweight. The purveyance of false promises from dietary supplements has been a major problem in recent times. I believe that most often, there is no bad intent, but there is excitement in new discoveries in natural medicine. Such excitement leads to premature conclusions on benefits of dietary supplements in some circumstances. While I am excited by the potential use of Hoodia gordonii as a revolutionary dietary supplement and as a starting substrate for the development of drugs for weight control, I believe that much further research is required.

The greatest acknowledgement must be made to the ancient tribe of the San bushmen of South Africa, who discovered the use of Hoodia gordonii as an appetite suppressant, perhaps thousands of years ago. The notion of "losing weight" never entered the mind of the primitive San bushmen. In these days of "nutritional colonialism" and global spread of western lifestyle, the health of many ethnic groups in third-world countries has become threatened. The urban areas of third-world countries are no longer typical of the traditions of these countries and South African native people have been downtrodden for many years. Fortunately, the San bushmen should benefit financially from the commercialization of Hoodia gordonii; and this will hopefully improve their lifestyle.

I wrote this book over my Christmas vacation in 2004. I felt there was an urgent need to review the subject of Hoodia gordonii which has been "pegged" as a major breakthrough in the management of healthy weight control. Therefore, this book is not a literary masterpiece, and I trust that it does not have too many rough edges. Among explosive interest in Hoodia gordonii rests a putative pathway to impact the global epidemic of obesity. Modern medicine waits with "baited breath" to watch the clinical outcome of the use of the "stinky" little plant called Hoodia gordonii. This plant seems to carry one of the many miracles of nature.

Stephen Holt, MD
January, 2005

FOREWORD

It is with utmost admiration that I write a foreword to this novel and new account of Hoodia gordonii. Stephen Holt, MD is a best-selling author with an unparalleled ability to synthesize information with meteoric speed. The succulent plant, Hoodia gordonii, became a focus of public interest in the latter part of 2004. In rapid response, Dr. Holt draws his writing gun from his holster to review the fascinating discoveries that surround Hoodia gordonii. With thousands of years of use of Hoodia gordonii in the food chain of South African natives, we are faced with the wisdom of ancient culture that discovered the ability of this plant to suppress appetite and thirst. The San bushmen of South Africa disclosed their secrets to western visitors in the 1930's; and South African researchers woke up to the importance of this finding in the 1960's when they commenced scientific studies on the biological effects of Hoodia gordonii in animals and humans.

As a practicing surgical gastroenterologist, with 40 years of clinical experience, I have treated thousands of people with weight problems. In my career, I have witnessed a rapid expansion of the human waistline in western society. Obesity is a very difficult disorder to manage, and no single diet has resulted in continued weight control in a significant number of people. Modern research points to the complexity of weight gain and weight loss must be considered a complex task. With failing interest in many fad diets, obese individuals have become increasingly desperate for new developments in weight control tactics.

Many dietary supplements and drugs used for weight control possess disadvantages or limitations. The desperate nature of the obese person is fueled by the realization that obesity is rapidly becoming the number one preventable cause of premature death and disability in western society. This has resulted in increasing popularity of more invasive ways of controlling weight, such as the use of gastric bypass surgery and its variations. Clearly, surgery is not generally attractive and it is not an option for everyone who is obese.

Hoodia gordonii carries a special promise for appetite control and decreased calorie intake, with resulting weight loss. Much further research is required to confirm the promises of Hoodia gordonii. This botanical or its extracts seem to be a valuable adjunct to behavior modification, lifestyle change, and exercise for effective weight control. The reported effects of Hoodia gordonii and extracted steroidal glycoside molecules on weight control seem too good to be true. However, emerging science seems to support the serendipitous observations of the ancient San bushmen. The bushmen used Hoodia gordonii to allay their intense feelings of hunger as they traveled through the deserts of South Africa where food and water are often scarce.

I find the contents of this book fascinating and Dr. Holt is appropriately cautious in his opinion about Hoodia gordonii, as an advance in effective, healthy, weight loss tactics. That said, his excitement for this new development in the fight against the worldwide epidemic of obesity shines through this book. The medical community is intrigued by what appears to be one of many "Natures' imprints" that can help with the obesity pandemic.

T.V. Taylor, MD
Clinical Professor, University of Texas
and Baylor College of Medicine, Texas
January 2005

TABLE OF CONTENTS

SPECIAL NOTE TO THE READER

This book is focused on a discussion of the use of the putative weight loss aid Hoodia gordonii, when taken as a food supplement. There is no intention to use this book as labeling for any dietary supplement. Before any person self-medicates, they should educate themselves. Anyone wishing to take Hoodia supplements should check with a health-care practitioner in any case of doubt. The self medication of established diabetes mellitus is not recommended. This book does not support a specific product for sale. The promise of Hoodia gordonii is very real, but it should be interpreted in the perspective of diet, drug and supplement failures for weight control.

INTRODUCTION

Hoodia gordonii is a "stinky" plant from South Africa with "miraculous properties". This cactus-like plant contains substances that may exert dramatic control over hunger, appetite, and thirst. Although the Hoodia gordonii plant looks like a cactus, it belongs to a category of plants called succulents. The use of Hoodia as an appetite suppressant is supported by colorful folklore history and recent scientific studies. Hoodia is well known to the San bushmen of South Africa, who learned to eat this plant to reduce hunger sensations from the teachings of their forefathers. The San bushmen of South Africa believe that Hoodia is their food, water, and medicine.

The Hoodia plant grows in the Kalahari desert region of South Africa, including Namibia, Angola, and Botswana. History records that the San people of the Kalahari desert used the Hoodia plant to reduce hunger and thirst when they traveled across the desert. This nomadic, ancient group of people was often deprived of food on long hunting expeditions in the desert, and famine was common. In 1937, a Dutch anthropologist discovered the traditional use of the Hoodia plant by the San bushmen, but this discovery lay fallow for many years. The folklore use of Hoodia represents one of nature's forgotten miracles, where the needs of a local population were served by one of "nature's imprints" in plants.

The majority of the populations in South Africa have looked for ways to sustain their nutrition, rather than suppress their appetite and lose weight. The 1960's witnessed the emergence of obesity as a global epidemic, and this prompted scientists in the South African government to pursue research on Hoodia as a novel, natural way of suppressing appetite, for weight control. The research was timely, as the city-dwelling South African developed a problem with obesity and obesity-related disease, just like many other industrialized countries. When the South African Council for Scientific and Industrial Research (CSIR) began testing the properties of Hoodia in 1996, they were amazed by

its effects as an appetite suppressant in animals and recognized imme-
diately its vast untapped potential in the fight against obesity.

While it is clear that the effects of Hoodia have been known for centuries by the San bushmen of South Africa, big business interests have
rushed recently to patent components of this plant for commercialization as a drug or food additive. The San bushmen have lived in the desert
regions of South Africa for at least 20-30,000 years and they have laid claim
to the use of Hoodia for appetite suppression as their own intellectual
property. Not only have the San (San bushmen) chewed the Hoodia plant
to suppress hunger and thirst, these native people have used the plant as
a primary food source when other foods were in scarce supply. The San
bushmen named the Hoodia gordonii botanical, as '*!khoba*' or '*Xhoba*'.

Following the initial research findings with Hoodia, it did not take
long for the researchers at CSIR in South Africa to interest other scientists in the potential use of Hoodia as an apparent, safe appetite suppressant. Government researchers in South Africa negotiated with the
biotechnology industry to license rights on patents for the use of extracts
from Hoodia. The idea was that Hoodia could form the basis for drug
development. Independent confirmation of the appetite suppressant
effects of Hoodia in animals and humans has piqued the interest of
Fortune 500 pharmaceutical and food companies.

The idea that one could be in possession of a safe appetite suppressant was seen by the pharmaceutical industry as a potential multi-
billion dollar windfall. While scientists and big business negotiated their
newfound commercial prospects, the downtrodden bushmen of South
Africa hired an accomplished South African attorney to protest the filing of patents on what they considered to be their own discoveries. The
"long arm of the law" has made many businessmen rethink the "Hoodia
circumstances" and the overall validity of the patents have been questioned from a number of perspectives. Holders of the patents on Hoodia
appear to have negotiated royalty payments to the San bushmen who
may become new-found millionaires, but the promises of Hoodia must
be fulfilled for this economic reward.

It is clear that there was widespread knowledge of the ability of
Hoodia gordonii to suppress appetite even prior to its "discovery" by
a Dutch scientist in 1937. Such widespread knowledge and open disclosure of the ability of Hoodia to have such effects on appetite, must
raise the question of whether or not a "use patent" on the Hoodia plant

could be valid. In this case, there was prior art, meaning widespread knowledge of the use of Hoodia as an appetite suppressant.

The biotechnology and pharmaceutical industry were planning to make drugs out of specific components of Hoodia gordonii (steroidal glycosides), but this approach, by using extracts of this plant, is not consistent with the traditional use of the whole Hoodia plant. While one must anticipate that business interests will try to protect patents, Hoodia gordonii has emerged recently in several dietary supplement markets as a natural product that is believed, by many, to be able to be sold without encumbrance. Time will tell. Upon information and belief, Hoodia is considered food in South Africa and "food" is difficult to patent.

In this book, the scientific evidence that exists in animals and humans to support Hoodia gordonii as an adjunct to weight control, is presented in detail. I admit that the information may be incomplete. When big business wants to commercialize a drug or a food component, open disclosure of scientific findings does not occur early in the development process. Scientific studies exist on components of Hoodia, indicating that it has direct effects on the central nervous system. In simple terms, Hoodia works by making people feel full after ingesting this plant with their diet. There is reported research in which Hoodia may have lowered food intake by a factor of up to fifty percent in both animals and humans.

When South African scientists first tested the Hoodia plant, they discovered that the plant contained previously unknown molecules that act on the brain (hypothalamus) to fool the body into "thinking" that food requirements have been satisfied. This sense of "feeling full" is due to the brain being tricked into believing that "satiety" exists. Satiety is a sense of fullness to the point of excess and "to satiate" is to satisfy fully or to excess, in a context most often related to food intake.

The body has complex mechanisms of controlling hunger or appetite and promoting feelings of satiety. In the case of Hoodia, it would appear that its mechanism of action is a direct effect on the central nervous system, probably as a result of its content of a group of compounds called steroidal glycosides or cardenolides. One of the real advantages of Hoodia is that it does not contain dangerous stimulant substances, unlike many other known appetite suppressants. Appetite suppression with "stimulants" has not been shown to be generally safe.

It appears that no serious or harmful side effects of Hoodia gordonii have been reported. Furthermore, its presence in the African food chain for many years provides a reasonable precedent of safety. While the safety of Hoodia gordonii, used in its naturally occurring form, may be reasonably assumed, one cannot assume that specific extracts of Hoodia or isolated molecules found in Hoodia (steroidal glycosides) may be safe. Research has not yet satisfied the question whether or not ingredients in Hoodia, other than the alleged active substances (steroidal glycosides), are responsible for its appetite suppressing effects. Hoodia gordonii contains variable amounts of antioxidants, fiber, organic material, together with biologically active substances such as sterol glycosides. Are there other active phytochemicals in Hoodia?

Interested scientists and the general public do not have all of the information on the science of Hoodia, due to lack of disclosure and the fact that the biological effects of Hoodia gordonii remain underexplored. It has been reported variably that one synthetic molecule produced by a pharmaceutical company, that resembled an active constituent (steroidal glycosides) within Hoodia, had little effect on appetite suppression, in comparison to the use of the natural compounds found in Hoodia gordonii. These circumstance ignited intense interest in the scientific community, because it may be that the real benefits of Hoodia may be best obtained from Hoodia in its natural form, rather than in the form of a synthetic extract.

Nature is very clever and it is not readily amenable to a quick copy of its biologically active compounds by synthetic chemistry. The pharmaceutical industry will not be able to use the naturally-occurring appetite-suppressing molecules found in the whole Hoodia plant, because there is just not enough Hoodia gordonii to supply the perceived need for a drug; and it may be that there is not enough Hoodia to go around as a supplement. These are key problems facing the use of Hoodia or its components for weight control. At the time of writing, the South African government has reported that the demand for Hoodia is rapidly outstripping its supply.

Hoodia has emerged as a new and powerful nutritional supplement that may suppress the body function of appetite expression. It is believed that Hoodia works by stopping cravings for food. It would appear that Hoodia is safe when used in its natural form, and the only reported side-effects of Hoodia appear to be its ability to energize, and its potential actions as a mild aphrodisiac or antidepressant.

Stephen Holt MD, January 2005

CHAPTER 1:

WHAT IS Hoodia?

Introduction

While obesity reaches epidemic proportions, the afflicted become increasingly desperate to find new ways to control body weight. The plant Hoodia gordonii (Hoodia) has been described as a "natural miracle" because it contains substances that suppress appetite. Hoodia and its constituents provide great promise for controlling calorie intake in the diet – a key factor in the control of body weight. The interest in Hoodia as a dietary supplement for weight control can only be described as explosive. Following major sales of Hoodia as a dietary supplement in Western Europe, Hoodia gordonii has recently become the focus of great interest among Americans. This interest was fueled by TV coverage of Hoodia in the famous documentary programs "60 Minutes" and "20/20". Following the airing of these TV shows, many articles have appeared in the press, drawing attention to the newfound use of Hoodia gordonii.

Hoodia: Botanical information

The potential of Hoodia gordonii as an aid for weight control has produced frenetic interest in this previously, little-known plant. Along with any strong, new interest in healthcare, public confusion often prevails. Hoodia gordonii has been incorrectly referred to as a cactus. While it has a prickly green appearance, like a cactus, it belongs to a group of plants called succulents of the *Asclepiadaceae* family. There are at least 2,000 species of the Asclepiadaceae group of plants, and half of these species are succulents. Succulent plants imply that the body of the plant is full of juice and has fleshy tissues that will conserve water. Breaking the skin of the plant Hoodia results in the flow of juices and presentation of "plant flesh". This material has been considered to be very nutritious by the San bushmen of South Africa. Although a variety of species of Hoodia are found in the desert regions of South Africa (Kalahari, Botswana, and Namibia), not all varieties of Hoodia have been used as appetite suppressants. The principal, prized plant of the bushmen is Hoodia gordonii.

There may be more than 20 different species of Hoodia that grow in short clumps with a vertical stem that is pale green in color. Attempts to farm the species Hoodia gordonii outside its normal habitat have been generally unsuccessful, with notable exceptions. Hoodia plants are extremely difficult to grow, and they need a lot of care and attention, with obligatory requirements of watering, sunlight exposure, and specific seasonal temperatures. It is important to understand these botanical facts, because a rush to use Hoodia could place this plant under great pressure and risk of extinction. The good news is that the South African government has controlled the supply of Hoodia; and they have strict criteria on harvesting programs that occur only at limited times during the year. Unfortunately, a drought was reported in some areas of the Northern Cape of South Africa in late 2004 and Hoodia production in the early part of 2005 could be compromised.

Some Hoodia plants are quite common, but Hoodia gordonii is the specific species that exhibits appetite suppressing effects. Although Hoodia plants are readily available for purchase for home gardens, most are not the species "gordonii". Hoodia plants are quite slow growing and having sampled the flesh of the Hoodia plant, I can report that it has an extreme bitter taste. Hoodia plants are known to produce flowers that have an unpleasant smell that attracts a variety of insects. The attraction of flies by the flowers of Hoodia gordonii is important in their cross pollination. It is stated, but not verified, that a Hoodia gordonii plant needs to be at least five years old before it develops enough biologically active compounds (sterol glycosides) to suppress hunger.

Hoodia gordonii is now grown from seedlings on approved farms in South Africa, and many of these farms have used the knowledge and wisdom of the San people in their commercial growing processes. The sale of authentic Hoodia gordonii will result in direct economic benefit for the San bushmen, who are a tribe that have major problems with adaptation to modern ways of life. I raise the issue of "authentic" Hoodia gordonii because fake material may be used in cheaper products labeled as Hoodia. Some material has been and will be sold as Hoodia gordonii, without consideration of its origin, quality or purity. At the time of writing, pure Hoodia gordonii bulk material from South Africa rose on average by one hundred dollars per kilo over a three-day period (late

December 2004). Many suppliers of bulk Hoodia gordonii material have been selling alleged extracts and whole powders of Hoodia gordonii, without providing certificates of authentication (www.hoodia-supreme.com, Hoodia Supreme™ is authentic Hoodia gordonii from South Africa). I cannot comment on other supplements.

Listening to the San Bushmen

Hoodia gordonii has been used for centuries by the San bushmen of South Africa. These people may have some times consumed Hoodia a couple of times a day on a regular basis. The "San" are known to have chewed on the plant during times of food scarcity, in order to alleviate hunger and thirst. Hoodia gordonii was found by bushmen to be particularly valuable for use during arduous hunting expeditions in the Kalahari desert. The Kalahari desert is a principle home for the San bushmen and it is a prime location for the growth of the succulent plant Hoodia gordonii.

The Kalahari is located near the Kgalagadi Transfrontier Park of South Africa. This desert region straddles the borders of the Republic of South Africa, Namibia, and Botswana. There are three main divisions of people within what is known overall as the "San culture". These divisions include the Khomani, the !Xun, and the Khwe. Understanding the distinction between different tribal groups within the "San culture" is quite difficult because of the use of indistinct terms that are not understood, except by local experts. For example, the term "Khwe" is used as synonymous with the label "San Bushman" in many circumstances. Other names are used to describe these people, e.g., "Basarwa" and "Kwankhala", but descriptive terminology changes with different geographic locations in the southern part of the African continent.

South Africa has many different tribal cultures. Since the collapse of apartheid there has been a systematic attempt to understand different social groups within indigent or indigenous populations. In a post-apartheid South Africa, the government is still sifting through different identities of subculture, as a prelude to defining the needs of different indigenous peoples. The San Bushman are a difficult group to identify as a homogenous social group. It would appear that the properties of Hoodia gordonii are known to several local tribesmen, perhaps even some tribes that may not be defined as San Bushmen per se. The power of this succulent plant, known to the "San" as *!khoba* (Hoodia) is going to be a continuing focus of international attention in the fight against the global pandemic of obesity. The world has finally listened to the "San people".

The San bushmen are a group of people that are threatened by the introduction of adverse lifestyle into their culture. It is reported that these people are beleaguered by wide spread substance abuse, with the use of marijuana and excessive alcohol consumption. The San are underprivileged and many have few possessions. The level of education among this nomadic population is poor and bushmen have entered urban areas without necessary skills to earn a living. The promise of Hoodia includes the possibility of economic support for the "San".

At one time, the San bushmen were positively persecuted by certain segments of South African society; and there is a hangover of opinion in South Africa that these people are not easily "absorbed" by modern society. It is pleasing to know that the post-apartheid government of Mandela and his colleagues were quick to recognize the needs of the San bushmen by granting them ownership of 150 square miles of land that has fine potential for the growth of Hoodia gordonii.

It should be understood that there has been some inconsistency in the reports of the use of Hoodia by modern San bushmen. One direct quote used in the media attributes the following statement to a member of the San bushmen tribe: *"I learned how to eat it* (Hoodia*) from my forefathers...It is my food, my water and also a medicine for me"*

While the San bushmen used Hoodia (Xhoba) for sustenance and survival at times of hunger, it is an alien thought to San bushmen that anyone would not want to eat! The traditional use of Hoodia by the San for appetite control is an enigma. While the San were staving off their hunger, they may have been altering their will to eat on occasion. It has been stated that the modern San bushmen may use Hoodia these days when a episodic obesity occurs in tribal members who have adopted western eating habits. It is clear that any modern reports of the folklore use of any herb or botanical can be subject to variable degrees of distortion. That said, the folklore use of herbs or botanicals is a platform to identify new treatments for disease.

The Modern Identity of Hoodia

Hoodia gordonii is emerging with a new identity, as it has started to promise a revolutionary approach to weight control. Following the initial discovery the use of Hoodia to suppress appetite by a Dutch visitor in 1937, it is reported that powdered Hoodia was stored in the laboratory of the Council for Scientific and Industrial Research (CSIR) of South Africa for years. In the 1960's, bright scientists at CSIR decided to study the effects of Hoodia on feeding habits in laboratory animals. Early scientific experiments showed that when laboratory animals were fed Hoodia, they reduced food intake and lost weight, without any signs of ill effects. In fact, the animals remained quite healthy, despite their voluntary reduction in food intake and weight loss that was attributed to the addition of Hoodia to their diet.

The CSIR, government researchers discovered that some specific extracts of Hoodia were active at suppressing appetite. They focused their attention on a group of molecules that are known as sterol glycosides. One of these molecules was particularly of interest because of its potent biological activity for the reduction of appetite. The CSIR in South Africa filed a patent in 1997 on the use of these previously unidentified Hoodia molecules (sterol glycosides). The rest is history when it comes to understanding the commercial importance of this discovery. The government researchers in South Africa did not synthesize the active molecules in Hoodia, but they isolated them in their natural forms.

In 1998, the CSIR of South Africa sold a license to their patent on Hoodia constituents to an English biopharmaceutical company called Phytopharm PLC (Cambridge, U.K.). In a game of "pass the parcel", the English biotechnology company attempted to sublicense the patent and the marketing rights to the "invention" to the Pfizer Corporation. This deal was reported to involve a 32 million dollar cash payment and a royalty stream. Around the time of this transaction legal problems started with the San bushmen and, upon information and belief, the Pfizer deal for Hoodia did not materialize?

First, there were problems in synthesizing sterol glycoside molecules that had the desired biological effect of appetite suppression. Reports emerged that synthetic molecules were tried and found not to be as effective as the naturally extracted molecules from the plant. Second, the CSIR faced an accusation from legal counsel of the San bushmen that they had sold rights in intellectual property that did not belong to them. Rhetoric ensued in the media in South Africa. The CSIR, as a government agency of South Africa, claimed (predictably) that they had the best interests of the San bushmen in their minds. That said, many people were puzzled by the initial exclusion of the San bushmen, in any attempt to commercialize their knowledge of the use of Hoodia. This dispute has placed the validity of certain patents in question. It is reported, but not easy to verify in detail, that the San bushmen had been awarded some financial compensation and some promise of future revenue from the use of Hoodia.

Contention Surrounding Commercial Rights to Hoodia

In a recent TV documentary "60 minutes", aired on the CBS TV channels, some of the contentions surrounding the commercialization of Hoodia were discussed. The TV correspondent, Leslie Stahl, of 60 Minutes visited South Africa and sampled Hoodia for herself. The TV footage was impressive. After grimacing, while chewing on a piece of Hoodia, Leslie Stahl reported her immediate loss of appetite. Back at the studio, a live interview occurred with the Chief Executive Officer of Phytopharm PLC, Dr. Richard Dixey. The interview was tense during the discussions of the rights of the San bushmen in the commercialization of Hoodia. Dr. Dixey claimed that he wanted to see the San bushmen share any profits that could come for the commercialization of molecules isolated from Hoodia. Dr Dixey is on record of having once reported that the San bushmen who discovered the value of Hoodia were no longer around. This is interpreted by some as an initial denial that the San bushmen should derive any benefit from the expected multi-billion dollar sales of drugs, created from copies of some of the naturally occurring compounds in Hoodia.

It appears that some kind of settlement had been reached between the San bushmen and the CSIR in South Africa in 2003. The magazine, Business Day reported in June 2003 that a royalty agreement had been offered to San bushmen, in the event that a new anti-obesity drug was developed from Hoodia research. One spokesmen for the CSIR implied that any profits would be shared equally with the San tribesmen and women, but what portion of all potential profits are to be shared remains unclear. The San bushmen must be grateful to their attorney, Roger Chennells, who fought loyally to obtain compensation for his clients. Mr. Chennells may be one of the attorneys who should be spared from

Shakespeare's aphorism about lawyers.

The popular TV show "20/20" echoed much of the content of the earlier "60 Minutes" TV broadcast. The "20/20" show aired in the U.S. in early January, 2005. However, the British Broadcasting Corp. (BBC) was first off the mark with a unique report about Hoodia gordonii and the San bushmen in the latter part of 2004. Tom Mangold, a correspondent for BBC2 television, traveled to Africa and sampled the appetite suppressing effects of Hoodia gordonii himself, and shared his experiences with his camera team. Tom Mangold reported a powerful "imagine this" story. He described the potential of an "organic pill", made from Hoodia, *that kills the appetite and attacks obesity*. Was he talking about a supplement, or a drug?

Mangold and his crew drove into the Kalahari desert, and found what they described as an *unattractive plant*, which was sprouting several tentacles, about the size of a large cucumber. These TV people discovered the unpleasant taste of Hoodia, and described their loss of appetite. The effects were almost immediate. After driving about four hours, back to Capetown, South Africa, from the desert, the TV crew reported that they did not even think about food, and that their *brains really were telling us we were full*, referring to themselves. Mangold described this as *a magnificent deception*. Later that day, none of the TV crew ate dinner, and no one in the group wanted breakfast. Mangold reported that the following day after eating Hoodia, he ate lunch without much appetite and without much pleasure. The TV personnel reported a gradual return of partial appetite, then full appetite, slowly, about 24 hours after they had eaten the "stinky, bitter-tasting plant".

The P57 Label of Phytopharm PLC

Phytopharm PLC has provided an arbitrary label for what they believed to be an active constituent of Hoodia. They have called the active molecule P57, because this was apparently the 57th active "biological" developed by Phytopharm PLC. While the emerging identity of the value of Hoodia in its clinical application has focused on drug development pathways, these avenues of development may not be ideal. First, there may be many different compounds in Hoodia that could work together in suppressing appetite when the plant is ingested in its natural form. Are sterol glycosides the only active constituents of Hoodia? The answer to this question remains to be determined.

Of course, there is a major disincentive for a pharmaceutical company to develop an anti-obesity drug from Hoodia if one can support the notion that the whole plant or its natural extracts are more effective than synthetic "drug" copies. This disincentive relates to the inability of anyone to make a plant "proprietary" or a plant extract "proprietary". In other words, anything that takes away the ability to legally control a product sale or distribution by a pharmaceutical or food company will defeat the omnipotence of "big business". In general, the pharmaceutical industry and the biotechnology industry will not invest money in any product, when they cannot derive exclusive, economic benefit.

Hoodia in Perspective:

What is Hoodia?

Hoodia gordonii is a succulent from a family of botanicals [Asclepiadaceae], with a spiny appearance resembling a cactus. Hoodia has been used for thousands of years by the San bushmen of South Africa, to control hunger and thirst during hunting expeditions in the Kalahari desert. Hoodia gordonii has piqued worldwide interest among doctors and scientists studying obesity, and has emerged as the focus of new methods to lower dietary calorie intake. Lowering calorie intake in the diet is perceived as the new revolution in sustained weight control, following disappointment with all fad diets for weight loss, including low-carb diets.

How does Hoodia work?

The media has exploded with reports of the miraculous benefits of Hoodia gordonii as simple, nutritional support for weight control. Hoodia gordonii has been featured on the internet, and in all public media, ranging from radio interviews through to newspaper reports. It is reported as beneficial weight control when used as a dietary supplement or in "drug research".

Where there is smoke, there is fire! Hoodia gordonii appears to contain substances that fool the brain into thinking that a person has eaten or is "full". The science supporting Hoodia's use is very strong. In fact, Hoodia has emerged as one of the best-selling dietary supplements in Western Europe, where fighting the flab is now as important as it is in the U.S.

The Science of Hoodia

Government researchers in South Africa have focused on compounds called sterol glycosides, present in Hoodia gordonii. Hoodia gordonii whole powder contains fiber, organic material, antioxidants and biologically active substances. The pharmaceutical industry has been so impressed by research findings with Hoodia gordonii that there have been multi-million-dollar deals to try and make drugs or food additives from constituents of Hoodia gordonii. Making a drug from Hoodia is not consistent with its traditional use as an appetite suppressant by native South Africans.

The consumption of Hoodia gordonii over thousands of years by the San bushmen creates a great precedent for the safety of the Hoodia plant, but it does not create precedence for the safety or effectiveness of a "drug derivative". Hoodia does not contain dangerous stimulant molecules, but it does contain substances that may mimic the effects of glucose on nerve cells in the brain. Controlled clinical and laboratory experiments show much promise of Hoodia for weight control. Some experiments have shown that obese people taking Hoodia have reduced their calorie intake by an amazing amount of one thousand calories per day.

Hoodia Matches the Key Public Health Initiatives

Two thirds of all Americans are overweight. Weight control requires a firm resolution of a well-planned diet, with calorie control, and exercise. Obesity is often associated with high blood pressure, high blood cholesterol, and insulin resistance. This is the metabolic Syndrome X. This disorder affects 70 million Americans, and it is a common cause of premature disease and death.

Recent studies show that weight gain occurs over weekend and holiday excesses. Having a safe dietary supplement that can help to switch off appetite, or at least aid in control of appetite in a safe manner, is an outstanding new promise.

Chapter Summary

Hoodia gordonii was previously considered to be an uninteresting plant, from a relatively uninteresting habitat. There has been a renaissance of interest in the Hoodia family of succulent plants, given the demonstrated ability of this botanical to suppress appetite in an apparently safe and effective manner. Steeped in folklore history, Hoodia has emerged with strong scientific support for its beneficial effect in suppressing appetite. Weight control is only possible in the presence of behavior modification and healthy lifestyle, including exercise and control of calorie intake. Hoodia gordonii promises to be an effective way of curbing the appetite of many nations that are experiencing an ever increasing average weight and an expanding waistline.

The story of Hoodia is a prime example of how the folklore use of remedies of natural origin can form a basis for research that may often result in scientific breakthroughs. Most treatment approaches involve the proprietary interests of big business. Hoodia gordonii will become a dietary supplement of great interest worldwide, as there is increasing public knowledge of its apparently miraculous effects on appetite control. Nature is not easily fooled, even though Hoodia gordonii seems to fool the body by giving a sense of satiety (fullness).

CHAPTER 2

APPETITE CONTROL AND HOODIA

Understanding Energy Balance

Healthy people are able to maintain a steady balance of body energy over prolonged periods of time. Energy is taken into the body in the form of food, and this energy is used to support the chemistry of life. In addition, energy from food meets the needs of energy expenditure, as occurs during exercise. Nobody eats exactly the same amount of food every day, and therefore energy input into the body is somewhat variable. Eating small or large meal portions on different days makes body weight go up, or down, by a pound or so of body weight. Minor variations in body weight also occur by water gain or loss (a pint of water weighs about one and one quarter pounds).

While healthy people are able to maintain an energy balance, any major shift in the balance causes significant changes in body weight. This circumstance is a simple description of the laws of thermodynamics, where input of energy into the body (food) matches output of energy or use of energy by the body (e.g., body function or exercise). In fact, this is a description of the "energy equation" of the body.

Recent research has confirmed longstanding beliefs that the balance between energy into and out of the body does not match with perfection. This is because weight control depends on many different complex factors. One good example of the imperfect nature of this equation of "energy in and out of the body" is the observation that low carbohydrate diets can induce early weight loss, better than "regular diets" that contain the same amount of calories. In fact, this situation is what led to the popularity of low-carb diets. These diets cause early, accelerated weight loss in comparison to many other diets. The problem is that this weight loss is often short-lived and it is followed often by weight regain. Weight regain occurs when the individual does not stick carefully to the low-carb diet, if the low carb diet is discontinued, or if simple carbohydrates are introduced into the diet following an initial phase of low-carb dieting. Weight regain occurs in the majority of people after six or twelve months of a low-carb dieting spree. This circumstance has led to the partial "fizzling" of the "low carb craze".

Recent disenchantment with low-carb diets has been discussed in detail in the media, but carbohydrate restricted diets are certainly important and effective in causing short-term weight loss. The restriction of simple sugars in the diet is an important approach to managing pre-diabetes or the metabolic Syndrome X (affecting up to 70 million Americans) or Type II diabetes mellitus, which is the commonest form of diabetes (affecting about 20 million Americans). The U.S. epidemic of weight-gain is rapidly becoming the number one preventable cause of death and general disability in the population. Therefore, the "new revolution in diets" must focus on healthy weight control which involves many factors, other than a fad diet alone.

Forget Diets Alone

Controlling weight is very difficult for the average Western person, because of the widespread emergence of excessive calorie intake. In addition, the wrong kind of food, physical inactivity, and other adverse lifestyle factors cause weight gain. If the average American could avoid an obsession with fad diets, and focus on a more comprehensive approach to weight control, there would be major progress in controlling our expanding waistlines. This comprehensive approach must include: behavior modification, control of calorie intake, a reasonable level of exercise, and attention to factors that promote weight control, e.g, restful sleep, reduction of stress, and removal of substance abuse, including simple sugar (a substance of common abuse in western society).

There has been a recurrent, silly statement from some nutritionists, that *"calories don't count"*. In fact, this misguided notion was put into effect on several occasions in the past decade with the introduction of absurd ideas such as "lose weight while you sleep", "eat all you want and get thin", etc. Why does this kind of obvious gobbledygook appeal to anyone? The reason is obvious. People afflicted with overweight status, or obesity, are often desperate and will cling at any straw to lose weight.

Human nature directs us all to look for an easy way out of a problem, and the American consumer is still engaged in the mythical and magical thoughts that a weight-loss miracle exists on the horizon. It remains to be seen if Hoodia is this miracle? Weight control is a serious business requiring resolution and commitment. The time has come to take a couple of steps backwards, and look at weight management in a rational manner. One must use a scientific, evidence-based aproach to make good decisions about management of excessive body weight. Here endeth "the sermon", which may not be entirely good news for many people who have health-challenging stores of body fat. Please do not slam this book closed, Pandora's box has opened and hope remains!

More About Energy In and Out of the Body

Let's look at weight control as though it is a simple household budget. Being under- or overweight is the result of an imbalance in energy budgets. In general terms, the underweight person does not eat enough and the overweight person has eaten too much or eats enough to maintain their weight gain. "Staying fat" does often require high energy (food) intake. We talk about energy into the body, but the real discussion is the calorie intake, as a consequence of what kind of food and how much food a person eats. Bear in mind that energy balance determines weight, but energy cannot be subject to a touch or a feel, and "energy" has no weight, as such.

Back to the household budget, if you spend more money on your home than the amount of money coming into your home, you will draw upon your savings. Over a period of time you will run out of money as you cash in your savings. In similar terms, the amount of body fat you have is like your savings account, except its value is stored as energy. Energy stores in the body are mainly in the form of fat deposits which constitute an "ugly savings account". The savings account of fat can receive deposits, or withdrawals.

The "value" of the fat savings account depends on energy balance. This is the amount of food you consume (energy in), balanced by the amount of energy expenditure. It is very important for an individual to understand that the more energy expended from the body the more tendency there is to reduce fat deposits. Weight control must involve a situation where more energy is withdrawn from the body, and less energy is put into the body. Please remember that "energy", in our discussion, is the same as the amounts of food; and the types of selected food are important.

Food As Energy

If one was to take food and burn it, then it releases its energy. The body "burns" food to make energy. Different types of food contain different amounts of energy and the unit of energy is the calorie or kcal. The simplest way to arrive at the energy value of food is to calculate the number of calories that have come from proteins, fat, carbohydrate, and alcohol in the diet. The amount of calories present in different types of food should be memorized.

One gram of carbohydrate or one gram of protein contains about 4+ kcal. In contrast, one gram of fat contains 9 kcal. It may come as a surprise to many people that one gram of alcohol contains 7 kcal. To reinforce the importance of these "calorie values," one should appreciate that fat by weight contains more than twice the calories of carbohydrate or protein, by weight. This observation of the calorie density of fat, together with the knowledge that some types of fats are unhealthy, led to the "low-fat diet craze" of the 1980's. These days, we recognize that not all fat is bad and more recently we have begun to focus on the pre-existing knowledge that not all carbohydrate intake is bad. Let me explain.

Good Fats, Bad Fats: Good Carbs, Bad Carbs

The best diet contains a balance of carbohydrates, fat, and protein, without useless calories from alcohol. However, the circumstances are not quite so simple because we now recognize good carbohydrates and bad carbohydrates, in the same way that we have recognized good fats and bad fats. The terms "good" or "bad" refer to implications for general health. Good carbohydrates are those complex forms of carbohydrates that are most often found in fruits and vegetables, in association with other vital nutrients such as antioxidants. Fruit and vegetables also contain valuable types of soluble and insoluble fiber. Dietary fiber promotes general health in many ways.

It is quite confusing for many people to learn that fiber is often composed of carbohydrate units; but the carbohydrates in fiber are generally not absorbed into the body. Dietary fiber resists digestion by the human gastrointestinal tract, in its areas of maximum absorption of nutrients (the small intestines).

People are tired of being told that they do not eat enough fruits and vegetables, but standard advice for low carb diets often results in limitations in fruit and vegetable intake. This is an unhealthy part of "low carb dieting" for many people. A good intake of fruit, vegetables, dietary fiber, berries, nuts, and grains is known to be very healthy. While food scientists raise their voices about fruit and vegetable intake and its benefits for health, the U.S. nation continues to turn a deaf ear. Increasing fruit and vegetable intake could reduce the occurrence of many chronic diseases, including heart disease, inflammation, and cancer.

Imbalances in Body Energy

While as many as 500 million people worldwide are starving, the major problem in industrialized nations is overindulgence in too much of the wrong kind of food. Our biosphere is experiencing a major imbalance in food (energy) availability, while our bodies fight to maintain energy balance. In the first week of January, 2005, the USDA added some "cute", new recommendations to the "Food Pyramid Guide" by focusing on reduction of calorie intake in the American diet. I believe that the USDA should dismantle the "Food Pyramid" and start again.

Health and wellbeing demands balance in many domains of our lifestyles and our over–nutrition is precipitating a group of diseases of dietary excess. These diseases include obesity, Type II diabetes mellitus, hypertension and hyperlipidemias (high blood cholesterol).

While much focus is placed on obesity itself, it is the obesity-related or associated disorders that often result in premature death or disability. About 70 million Americans have the metabolic Syndrome X, where the obvious presence of being overweight is variably associated with high blood pressure and high blood cholesterol. These disorders are linked together by an underlying problem with the function of insulin, where the tissues of the body become resistant to the actions of insulin (insulin resistance).

The metabolic Syndrome X will be discussed in more detail later in this book. Syndrome X is the prime example of how being overweight causes metabolic disease. The widespread occurrence of Syndrome X affords a principal reason why one must consider weight gain as only one part of a constellation "ugly disease companions" that "hang together" and threaten our life.

Energy intake and food preferences are an important part of our understanding of the obesity epidemic and its associated disorders, such as Syndrome X. There are large differences in requirements of food (energy) intake from one person to the other. These differences in energy needs are caused by many factors, of which the most important include: age, gender, the amount of physical activity, etc. There is a measure of body fat used by scientists, called the fat-free body mass, which determines energy needs. If one looks at the combined influence of fat free body mass, age and sex, together, one can explain the bulk of the differences that exist among people, in terms of their resting metabolic rate.

Metabolic Rate of the Body

The resting metabolic rate relates to energy burned in keeping the body "ticking over", with its normal chemistry of life. The chemistry of life needs energy to function effectively for health. While readers without a science background may be confused by terms, the resting metabolic rate is simply a measure of the energy expended by the body to maintain its own basic functions and internal balances (homeostasis). One simple analogy would be the amount of energy or food required to keep the body "ticking over", like a car engine running while stationery.

The stationary car needs energy (gasoline) to run while stationary, but much less gasoline is required for the stationary, idle engine than the engine action that creates motion for the car. People in western nations are becoming quite idle. This means that the resting metabolic rate in humans is very often the greatest contributor to total daily energy expenditure of the human body! Furthermore, the more idle the "running automobile" or the living human body, the more the resting metabolic rate is the greatest contributor to energy expenditure. In our idle Western society, our resting metabolic rate is emerging as our only way of burning energy.

Understanding these basic principles must help people to understand how lack of exercise is sending our energy equation "out of whack"; and it is pushing us to a state of fat storage (energy storage), resulting in obesity. There are many factors that cause the body to develop an "overweight status" and even more factors that act to cause a perpetual state of obesity. If only one message can be made clear, it is the amount of food and the type of food eaten that are very important factors in controlling weight gain and obesity.

Eating Beyond Our Appetite

The amount of food we eat is often a function of our appetite, or our ability to eat beyond signals that tell us that we are full (satiety signals). The importance of appetite suppression in weight control is increasingly apparent and the makes the promise of Hoodia very enticing.

Cutting down on energy input into the body (calories in food) will do much to help control body weight. This discussion is very relevant to the new discovery of Hoodia, as a potential way of assisting in cutting down energy (calories) intake in the diet. Before we can discuss the science of Hoodia, it is important to understand how the body controls our eating habits. These habits control our food (energy) intake. We are all aware of the powerful drive of hunger and the satisfaction of feeling full after a meal. The human body has clever ways of controlling hunger, appetite and food intake.

Food preference and calorie intake are both important

There are studies in the medical literature which show that calorie counting in the diet may provide a disincentive for some people on a weight-reducing diet. In fact, it is difficult to run one's life by numbers and regimentation. With a little bit of practice, many people can look at any plate of food and estimate the number of calories in the meal. Simple skills at estimating calorie intake do not require detailed records of calorie counting, but some basic information about the food energy values should be committed to memory.

In simple terms a teaspoonful of table sugar contains 25 calories, whereas a teaspoonful of fat or oil contains 50 calories. An ounce of lean meat contains about 50 calories, but if the meat has a medium fat content, the calorie content increases to 75 calories per ounce. High fat meats such as bacon or marbled sandwich meats contain about 100 calories per ounce. One half of cup of average vegetables contains about 25 calories and a portion of unsweetened fruit contains about 50 calories. These numbers refer to modest portions. With this knowledge in mind, an important issue is to take a balanced amount of good fat, good carbohydrates and good protein in a meal that has a "reasonable portion size".

Skewed Ideas About Meal Portion Sizes

Unfortunately in America the average person's idea of a food portion size often represents an overindulgence. Appropriate meal portion sizes for a average meal need not be carefully calculated. I can give a good example of a simple approach for controlling dietary calorie intake. An optimum calorie-controlled meal, using a balanced diet for healthy people, may be something like a small baked potato, a four ounce fish fillet, one half a cup of green vegetables and a beverage that contains good nutrients, such as a glass of low fat milk. One important recent observation is the role of calcium within low fat diary products for helping with weight control. A suitable desert, in an ideal meal, would be yogurt without too much simple sugar, or substitution of sugar with a healthy, low-calorie sweetener. In fact, low fat yogurt has been shown to promote weight control in recent scientific studies.

Are All Dietary Calories Equal?

In the 1980's food scientists became obsessed with the idea that not all calories in various foods are equal in their contribution to fat storage by the body. Experiments did show variably that energy derived from fat in the diet was more "fattening" that energy derived from carbohydrate or protein in the diet. It was argued that when total calories in different types of foods are taken in equal amounts, the food that is higher in fat content contributes more to weight gain or obesity. From this scientific observation the "low fat food craze" emerged in the 1990's. The idea that fat in the diet was the real "miscreant", when it came to weight gain, has been questioned over the past few years by scientists who support the low carbohydrate diet approach. I have discussed these matters in detail in my book "Enhancing Low Carb Diets" (www.wellnesspublishing.com)

Simple Sugar: a Dietary Miscreant

There has been a missing–link in thoughts about weight control. Scientists have confirmed that carbohydrate restriction in the diet with liberal fat content can caused accelerated short term weight loss (e.g. The Atkins diet). These observations created much confusion for diet enthusiasts and even more confusion for some medical professionals. The body is very clever at handling food preferences and energy needs. When excessive fat is taken in the diet, without carbohydrate, the body switches its chemistry to promote a variable state of "Ketosis". The switch of body metabolism to ketosis contributes to weight loss, at least by depressing appetite, or by the diet itself causing an overall reduction in calorie intake!

Why Did the Low Fat Diet Craze Fail?

In the early 1990's American consumers were faced with a vast selection of low fat foods in supermarkets. The big problem with weight control and low fat foods related to the substitution of carbohydrates for fats in many foods. In many cases, low fat foods were loaded with simple sugars. While many people had focused on the idea that dietary fat was the cause of nation's weight gain, less focus was directed to the importance of simple sugar, causing insulin responses in the body that lead to weight gain. When one takes simple sugars in the diet, blood glucose tends to rise quickly and blood insulin "surges" occur. Over time, the body tissues may develop a resistance to insulin and the body develops a tendency to pour out more insulin to control upward swings in blood glucose (sugar). Insulin is a powerful signal to the body to cause fat storage.

While insulin is important in lowering blood sugar, the hormone insulin has many effects on the body. I reiterate that insulin is a powerful signal to the body to cause fat storage. In addition, excess insulin may tend to cause raises in blood pressure and abnormalities in blood cholesterol. In simple terms, this is the way that excess simple sugar intake tends to operate as a major factor in the development of the metabolic Syndrome X.

The metabolic Syndrome X will be discussed in detail later in this book; but within the metabolic Syndrome X, a constellation of health-challenging problems occur together. These problems include obesity or overweight body status, combined variably with high blood pressure and high blood cholesterol. This constellation of problems is linked together by underlying insulin resistance and insulin excess in the body, each of which is caused to major degree by excessive sugar intake in the diet. I want to purposely reiterate the health challenges of the metabolic Syndrome X.

The preceding information means that the promises of a low fat diet for weight control were false promises, largely because many low fat foods were high calorie, sugar-containing foods. In fact, many low fat foods were quite delicious and they appealed to the common "sweet taste" preferences of Americans. It is known that many Americans have a "sweet tooth". There is a tendency for consumers to think that low fat foods mean low calorie foods and this results in many people eating excessive amounts of low fat foods, with the mistaken idea that they are "dieting". The USDA Food Pyramid Guide compounded false beliefs in good food selection, by recommending too much refined carbohydrate in the diet. The pendulum of opinion swung in the opposite direction in the late 1990's, when the nation embraced "the low carb craze".

Why is the Low Carb Craze Failing?

There are a number of reasons why the "low carb craze" is losing popularity. I forecasted the failure of the frenetic interest in low carb diets in my book titled "Enhancing Low Carb Diets" (2003, www.well-nesspublishing.com). In fact, there is not a diet known to medicine that has resulted in sustained weight loss. The reader should reflect on this statement and I propose that this is "matter of fact". These matters of fact apply to the "low fat craze" and they apply to any other "fad diets". It is clear that weight control involves more than diet alone. While a diet involving calorie control and the correct selection of food groups are important in weight control, weight loss is a function of many factors, including behavior modification, exercise and a healthy lifestyle.

American healthcare consumers have been thoroughly confused about this or that diet! Low carb diets, such as the Akins diet or the South Beach Diet, do cause short term weight loss for a variety of reasons. One reason is quite obvious to many food scientists, but it may not be obvious to the average person who is trying to lose weight. A low carb diet will cause accelerated weight loss due to water loss from the body, but it does also cause early fat loss in many people.

One reason for the short term effectiveness of low carb diets is that people on such diets are excluding carbohydrates from their diets; and the average American may take more than half of their daily calories from carbohydrates. Thus, a low carb diet is a form of "forced calorie control". Furthermore, excessive protein and fat in a diet will reduce the appetite of many people, as a result of the frequent switch of body chemistry towards circumstances called "ketosis". A body status of "ketosis" causes appetite loss.

I believe strongly that the restriction of simple carbohydrate in the diet is a step in the right direction, in moving to an optimum diet for weight control. Remember diets often need tailoring to individual needs. A muscular teenager needs more food than a sedentary worker. My strong belief in simple sugar restriction in diets is based on the fact that as many as 70 million Americans may have insulin resistance. Resistance to the effects of insulin requires some degree of restriction of simple sugars in the diet. Robert Atkins, MD and others stated consistently that a low carb diet can overcome insulin resistance. This is not consistently the case. While restriction of simple sugars is an important step in controlling weight gain and the metabolic Syndrome X, it is not the whole story.

These are some of the reasons why I wrote the book entitled "Enhancing Low Carb Diets" (www.wellnesspublishing.com). Furthermore, this is the reason why I introduced the concept of the need to facilitate the actions of a carbohydrate restricted diet. However, I do believe that complex carbohydrates form an important part of a calorie control diet and these types of carbohydrates are most often found, along with dietary fiber, in fruits and vegetables. Many people who stuck to an Atkins diet were strangers to fruits and vegetables and, in some respects, this is what made the copycat "South Beach Diet" generally more acceptable, but no more effective!

Understanding Hunger, Appetite, and Satiety...

The amount of food that someone eats and their selection of different types of foods are controlled by clever body and brain functions. These mind and body (mindbody) functions are influenced greatly by social and behavioral factors. Indeed, hunger and appetite are controlled in a complicated manner by many body signals and brain functions. The overall combination of these complicated body functions work to balance energy storage by the body (fat deposits), with the intake of energy in the form of food.

These energy-balancing processes are also influenced by energy expenditure from the basic chemistry of life (metabolic rate) and exercise. It is important to have a basic understanding about the role of hunger, appetite and satiation in the control of energy balance or imbalance. Energy imbalance most often results in obesity in western society, but reductions of energy input into the body can result in weight loss.

It is useful to make some basic definitions of the terms: hunger, appetite and satiety, in order that they can be clearly distinguished by the reader. Hunger is a sensation that forces a need for someone to eat. Hunger will cause food-seeking behavior. When hunger is experienced as a strong desire, it can result in very negative and unpleasant sensations. We have learned that the San Bushmen of South Africa dealt with their unpleasant sensations of hunger by using the Hoodia plant. In contrast, appetite is best described as a desire to eat which is often accompanied by feelings of hunger. Unlike hunger, appetite is by itself considered by most people to be a pleasant sensation. It would appear that Hoodia is able to make appetite go away to a major degree.

The word "satiety" refers to a feeling of fullness or satisfaction, most often experienced after a meal. A feeling of satiety acts as a prompt or signal to make people stop eating. However, many people can learn easily to eat beyond their own feelings of satiety. The pleasure of eating can override feelings of fullness in "social gluttons". Almost everyone has eaten beyond their level of satiety and such people can easily identify with their own dietary excesses. It may surprise many readers to know that how the actual origin of feeding behavior is initiated remains somewhat a scientific mystery.

If an individual keeps eating beyond their satiety level then they can dampen their feelings of fullness. Some, but not all people, who are overweight have learned to repeatedly eat beyond a level of satiety, or simply "pig-out". Many of my friends and I have "pigged-out" on social occasions, without understanding that repeated overeating results in cumulative weight gain. Recent scientific studies show that weekend food binges and holiday excesses result in both temporary and cumulative weight gain and that most people cannot lose the weight that they accumulate on festive occasions. Therefore, our short-lived dietary excesses contribute greatly to our cumulative weight gain as a nation.

Body Regulation of Hunger and "Feeling Full" (Satiety)

The body has several ways of helping its own energy balance. This means that the healthy body tends to resist storing too much energy (fat deposits). Body mechanisms that control energy intake (food) are very intelligent and they must help in "decisions" on how often and how much people should eat. The many signals that tell the body to engage in measured food intake act mainly through body sensations of hunger and satiety. These sensations are controlled by a special portion of the brain called the hypothalamus.

When healthy people are free to make food choices, body controls work with consistent accuracy. Hunger seems to be a survival instinct and it is "in–born" in all creatures. Hunger makes us eat to live, but appetite is more of a learned response to food.

Many people can experience appetite without any feelings of hunger. This means that the pleasure of eating can be so appealing that it can occur for enjoyment alone. It is quite understandable why people can look for comfort in food, because eating is pleasurable. One may begin to see how complicated hunger and appetite may be. When one is engaged in pleasurable experiences, one can sometimes forget mild hunger and totally forget appetite! Equally, when an individual is placed under stress then they may not feel like eating. Anxious and worried people often lose their appetite, or some gain an appetite! This is feeding for comfort.

When the average person eats a good meal, their brain receives signals of satisfaction. Chewing and swallowing food delivers food that is accommodated by the stomach. These body events trigger satiety signals to the brain. These signals come from nerves that are activated in the digestive tract and messages from these nerves are relayed to the brain. For example, the stomach contains stretch-receptors which "fire signals" when the stomach expands due to an accumulation of food. In addition, the stomach and the digestive tract can release hormones that act as signals of satiety (e.g., cholecystokinin or CCK). Body hormones and nerve signals from the digestive tract can act on the central nervous system. These signals have special actions on the region of the brain called the hypothalamus. The hypothalamus controls sensations of hunger and satiety and acts as a "switch box."

Getting to Know the Hypothalamus of the Brain

The hypothalamus is a portion of the brain that receives many signals from different parts of the body. It receives messages about body temperature and body chemistry. This area of the brain also responds to the amount of nutrients entering the bloodstream. Blood sugar concentrations are measured by the hypothalamus. This sensing of blood sugar triggers a sensation of fullness (satiety). The role of the hypo-thalamus in controlling body functions has been well demonstrated in experiments where damage to this area of the brain has been found to cause major differences in eating habits and body metabolism. Damage to one area of the hypothalamus can cause overeating and damage to another area can cause under-eating. Animals with damage to various areas of the hypothalamus can become extremely obese or starve to death. The hypothalamus acts like a special controller of many body signals; and it directs the body to eat after it receives and analyzes much information from nerves and messenger molecules.

There are many other factors that are involved in hunger and appetite. Such factors range from influences in the environment, diseases, pleasure seeking, and even the taking of medications or dietary sup-plements. One big problem for overweight individuals is their inability to control their appetite. In addition some people crave certain kinds of foods, especially sweet or fatty foods. Modern research indicates the powerful behavioral effects caused by sugar in the diet. It appears that satisfying urges for sweet foods involves areas of the brain that control sensations of pleasure.

Just like the use of marijuana, or illicit drugs or alcohol, the brain of some people can develop a dependence on sugar. This is the basis of what some people have called "sugar addiction". The concept of car-bohydrate addiction seems to have supporting evidence in both animal and human scientific experimentation. When laboratory rats are fed excessive amounts of simple sugars which are then withdrawn from their diet, the rats exhibit symptoms and signs of withdrawal reactions. These reactions are quite similar to the withdrawal reactions that can be observed when drugs of addiction are stopped. There is a strong rea-son to believe that simple sugar is a substance of abuse. Therefore, "car-bohydrate addiction" appears to be a real phenomenon in some people. Table 1 lists many factors that can alter hunger and appetite:

HUNGER:

FACTORS CONTROLLING FOOD INTAKE	EXAMPLES
EMOTIONS	Thoughts, stressful events, mood etc.
BRAIN	Hypothalamic functions, other centers in the brain e.g. pleasure centers.
ENVIRONMENT	Social groups, peer-pressure, food availability, climatic conditions, exercise, etc
DISEASES	Metabolic Syndrome X, obesity, anorexia nervosa, diabetes mellitus, pre-diabetes, psychological problems, mental illness, etc.

APPETITE:

FACTORS CONTROLLING FOOD INTAKE	EXAMPLES
PLEASURE SEEKING	Good tasty food, good food texture, sugar content (sweetness), fat content (mouth feel)
DRUGS/SUPPLEMENTS	Illicit drug use, antidepressant drugs, appetite suppressing drugs or supplements, etc.
DISEASES	Cancer, inflammation, diabetes mellitus, etc.
SOCIAL ISSUES	Culture, habits, family pressure, etc.
MISCELLANEOUS	Body metabolism, hormones, specific appetites ("Sweet-tooth", "Salty-tooth", etc.), food aversions or food craving, climate, etc.

Table 1: This table illustrates many different factors that control or influence hunger and appetite. These factors work together to control the amount and type of food that people may eat. This list of influences on hunger and appetite is quite incomplete and each factor that controls food intake works through unique or combined mechanisms, involving nerves or messenger molecules. The end result is that the body works through some final pathway that represents an attempt to maintain an energy balance. It is apparent that medical, social, behavioral, and psychological factors operate to control hunger and appetite. One very important operating factor that controls food preference may be poverty. Financially underprivileged groups of society may be forced to eat cheap, junk food. In fact, improving general economic status in the U.S. has been proposed as a valid way of fighting the obesity epidemic.

CHAPTER 3

FAILURE OF DIETS ALONE

More About Good Carbohydrates and Bad Carbohydrates, or Good Fats and Bad Fats

There is increasing recognition of the role of the dietary intake of simple sugars in the precipitation of weight gain and its associated problems. These days, food scientists are thinking in terms of "good" carbohydrates [complex carbs] and "bad" carbohydrates [simple sugars]. For many years, nutritionists have distinguished "good" fats [unsaturated fats, e.g., Omega-3 fatty acids] from "bad" fats. Unhealthy fats include saturated fats or hydrogenated fats produced from treated vegetable oils. Chemical hydrogenation of vegetable oil makes solid fats (e.g., margarine). These hydrogenated fats contain trans-fatty acids which are damaging to health.

Refined carbohydrates (simple sugars) cause surges in blood insulin, and excessive simple sugar intake in the diet contributes to the widespread epidemic of insulin resistance. Insulin resistance contributes to the metabolic Syndrome X, where problems with the function of insulin contribute to obesity, high blood pressure, and high blood cholesterol. This constellation of problems in Syndrome X can occur in variable combinations. Excessive dietary intake of refined carbohydrates is a pivotal cause of the modern epidemic of the metabolic Syndrome X and Type 2 diabetes mellitus, but they are not the whole story.

The most popular, contemporary, low carbohydrate diet was described by Dr. Robert Atkins, MD, but his initial dietary recommendations were self-modified over a period of 30 years. Dr. Atkins' Diet was joined in recent years by other popular low carb diets, including but not limited to: "The Zone," "Carbohydrate Addict's Diet," "Sugar Busters Diet" and the neophytic or saprophytic recommendations of "The South Beach Diet."

Is One Diet Better Than the Other?

While arguments prevail that one low carb diet is better than the other, there is no real evidence that such differences exist. Certainly, recent studies published in the New England Journal of Medicine in 2003 served as a "wake-up call" for conventional medicine, when the Atkins' Diet was shown to be effective and reasonably healthy, at least in the short term. Contrary to popular belief, these studies did not openly endorse the Atkins' Diet. Weight regain with the Atkins' Diet occurs at six or twelve months, or so, in many people – a "yo-yo" effect. In fact, every diet described in the history of weight management has suffered from a lack of effectiveness for "long-term" weight control. I submit this again as matter of fact, contrary to prevailing propaganda.

I must continue to dismiss the myths that underlie fads and fallacies of weight control by dietary means alone. Diet is important for weight loss, but without behavior modification and exercise, there cannot be sustained weight loss. This is bad news for the "would-be dieter" who cannot make the commitment to long-term weight control. Notions such as *"eat what you want and get thin," "lose weight without trying"* and *"take this magic pill or dietary supplement to lose weight in a healthy and effective way"* are comments without much foundation.

Ugly Disease Companions of Obesity

In more than 30 years of clinical practice, I have never seen an individual with a significant degree of obesity who did not have at least one complicating obesity-related disorder. In other words, obesity does not present itself as a single medical problem for treatment. This is why weight control tactics must involve a global health initiative.

The modern epidemic of Syndrome X (the metabolic syndrome) has reinforced the idea that obesity, or an overweight status, cannot be addressed in isolation. Syndrome X is the variable occurrence together of high blood pressure, high blood cholesterol and obesity linked by insulin resistance. We have learned that the metabolic Syndrome X affects as many as one in four of the population (at least 70 million US citizens). Overcoming health problems in the management of obesity is only possible, in many circumstances, by overcoming Syndrome X. My comments are relevant to many overweight people in western nations and an increasing number in industrialized areas of third-world countries.

Syndrome X is Associated With Many Diseases

Syndrome X is believed to be caused by insulin resistance which occurs as a consequence of excess consumption of refined carbohydrates in the diet, poor nutrition, genetic tendencies and idleness, etc. Therefore, recommendations to "just lose weight" are fundamentally incorrect for the vast majority of people with significant degrees of obesity.

Make no mistake in understanding the metabolic Syndrome X. Within the constellation of problems in Syndrome X, there are major changes in body chemistry. These "chemical changes" result in the emergence of other diseases, including: cardiovascular disease, infertility, inflammatory diseases, Type 2 diabetes mellitus, polycystic ovary syndrome (PCOS), liver disease and even certain kinds of cancer. These circumstances present a unifying concept of disease which resulted in my attempts to rename this condition of the metabolic Syndrome X as Syndrome X, Y and Z... (Holt S, "Combat Syndrome X, Y and Z...," Wellness Publishing, Newark, New Jersey, 2002). I reiterate that being overweight or being obese is not a "simple, unitary disorder."

Comparing Weight Loss Diets

One must look very carefully at new studies that compare degrees of weight loss with different dietary approaches. Shocking as it may seem, there have been relatively few of these studies over the years, even though there have been strong claims for the benefit of one dietary approach for weight control versus another. Recent scientific information presented at an American Heart Association meeting in 2003 showed that four different popular diets resulted in approximately equal weight loss in the short term, but these popular diets had different approaches in terms of the dietary intake of fat, carbohydrate or protein. In other words, the "weight–control" diets had different components or ratios of macronutrients.

These recent studies involved comparisons among the Atkins' Diet (low carb, high protein), the Ornish Diet (low fat), the Weight Watchers Diet (calorie restriction) and the Zone Diet (low carb, focused on low Glycemic Index foods). In these studies, scientists from Tufts University in Boston studied 160 overweight or obese men and women, over a period of one year. The individuals who participated in the study were educated on the different diets by being encouraged to read the respective published books on the diet; and these participants received group classes to educate them on the respective diets (edutherapy).

Several outcomes were looked at during these research comparisons of different diets. The researchers made repeated assessments of compliance with the diet among the participants; and measurements were taken of body weight, blood pressure, glucose, insulin and cholesterol. These measurements were made at varying intervals during the study. The results of this study were fascinating.

After 12 months of study, all participants reduced their body weight to a variable degree and reduced their health risks for heart disease in a variable manner. The most successful approach for reducing the risk of heart disease was the Weight Watchers Diet, but most weight loss was experienced on the Ornish Diet. Reductions in risks of heart disease were somehwat modest, being in the order of 5% with the Ornish program and 15% with the Weight Watchers program.

The Ornish Diet seemed to have the best effects on reducing bad cholesterol (LDL), whereas the Weight Watchers Diet and the Zone had less effect on this risk factor for heart disease. It was noteworthy that the Atkins' Diet did reduce bad cholesterol levels by about 8.6%. This finding is in keeping with other recent studies, where the Atkins' Diet has been shown to have no significant negative impact on levels of bad cholesterol in the blood (LDL) in the "short term", despite its high fat content. I reject the construct of this research in relatively small groups of patients, because it serves to foster the competitive mentality among different diets. All diets, used alone, will fail with time!

An Unreasonable Weight Loss Target?

People who want to lose weight often "start–off" with an unreasonable expectation about how much weight they can lose. The aforementioned studies by the Rutgers group of researchers showed that the people on the various diets lost an average of only 10 to 12 pounds, approximately. This was equivalent to only about 5% of their body weight. What was most striking was the major variation in the ability of people to stick to each type of diet. About one-third of people on the Weight Watchers or the Zone diets dropped out of the studies, but 50% of people dropped out of the Atkins and Ornish diets. This is somewhat surprising, since the Atkins' Diet has a reputation for being easy to comply with over a period of time, at least in contrast to many other diets.

Low Carb Diets Do Not Overcome Insulin Resistance

One might imagine that insulin resistance or a compensatory, excess circulating level of insulin may be overcome by low carb diets. After all, it is the appearance of glucose in the blood that drives the body to secrete insulin. However, low carb diets do not overcome insulin resistance to a major degree. Modern research shows that any improvements in insulin resistance are related to the weight loss induced by a diet, rather than the elimination of dietary carbohydrates alone. I have repeated these facts, so that readers may understand the inadequacies of "low carb diets" alone for many people who have co-existing metabolic Syndrome X.

Diet Confusion

There has been massive public confusion about the best approach to weight control. This confusion has revolved largely around recommendations for "this or that kind of diet." A few years ago, the USDA assembled a few "diet gurus," including Dr. Atkins, to discuss the pros and cons of various diets. A "free for all" debate ensued and the public was left with more confusion than they had prior to the proceedings. From the confusion, I see advantages in reducing simple sugar intake, but I see less advantage with the reduction of complex carbohydrate intake, especially because complex carbohydrates are basically found in the fruit and vegetable component of a healthy diet. Eliminating fruit and vegetable intake in the diet cannot be considered healthy.

I am convinced that simple sugars are the miscreant for many overweight people in America, but perhaps not for all. One thing is clear, that without calorie restriction, behavior modification, exercise and change from adverse lifestyle to positive lifestyle, there can be no impact on the pandemic of obesity. The diet gurus all agreed that calories in the diet "do count," except perhaps Dr. Atkins.

Obesity: A Problem for the US Nation and a Global Epidemic

Some soothsayers tell us that by the year 2050, almost every American will become overweight. This horrifying projection is based on the assumption that the occurrence of obesity will increase at its current level. Perhaps we have tended to focus on the cosmetic aspects of obesity. These social issues surrounding obesity may precipitate a degree of embarrassment or even shame for some people. These are not constructive thoughts. The real significance of obesity to Western nations and some Third World countries is the occurrence of many obesity-related diseases, together with associated, mounting death rates.

While as many as 70 million Americans are overweight and 50 million are obese, there are about 1.7 billion people worldwide who share these traits. Weight gain has emerged as a global problem; and it is a universal risk to health. Europeans have commented on the "fattening of America" in many contexts, but at least one in five Europeans are obese and perhaps 35-40% are overweight? Obesity contributes to about 300,000 deaths in the US on an annual basis, whereas it causes about 30,000 deaths in the UK.

There seems to be a need to redefine what constitutes an overweight status for some nations. According to the World Health Organization, lesser degrees of being overweight are associated with illness and death in some Asian countries. Americans can see its "nutritional colonialism" and exported lifestyle at work to produce a global pandemic of obesity.

Obesity, Syndrome X,
Pre-Diabetes and Type 2 Diabetes

Before one starts to assess the overall negative effects of obesity and its related disorders, one must understand the relationship between obesity and the modern epidemic of diabetes mellitus. There are 70 million Americans who have a condition called the metabolic syndrome or Syndrome X (Figure 1). Syndrome X requires careful definition and description, if the real advantages of carbohydrate restriction in the diet can be fully appreciated. Syndrome X is a combination of factors which are almost invariably associated with an overweight status. I repeat, again, the simplest definition of Syndrome X as the variable combination of obesity, high blood pressure and high blood cholesterol, all linked by resistance to the hormone insulin. (Figure 1)

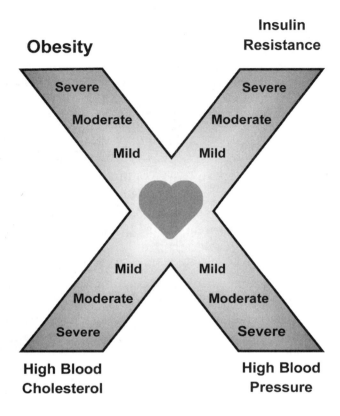

Figure 1: The multidimensional components of Syndrome X which account for cardiovascular risks. **Note:** Each component can be variably present and the manifestations of this disorder are protean (many and complex).

Insulin Resistance

Insulin is known to push glucose into tissues of the body, where it is used as fuel for the chemistry of life. Insulin resistance occurs when the body does not take the command of insulin. When insulin resistance is present, the body reacts by making more insulin and so insulin levels become high in the blood. This is the underlying problem that generates the combination of problems found in Syndrome X. While we all recognize the ability of insulin to help the body handle glucose, it is not quite as apparent to many individuals that insulin in excess can give signals to body organs to make them function in a negative manner for health.

Insulin's Actions: Beyond Glucose Handling

Insulin gives prime signals to fat cells to store fat. Hence, obesity goes hand in hand with insulin excess and resistance in many people. Insulin can tell the liver to make cholesterol and it can tell tissues of the body to raise blood pressure. One can now see, in somewhat simplistic terms, why obesity, high blood pressure and high blood cholesterol occur together under the umbrella terms "Syndrome X" or "the metabolic syndrome". Furthermore, insulin can tell the ovaries to secrete male-type hormones, tell the body to make inflammatory messenger molecules and even tell genetic material to express cancer growth. Thus insulin resistance and excess causes a diverse array of diseases (Syndrome X, Y, and Z…).

The Concept of Syndrome X, Y and Z…

I reiterate that Syndrome X is even more diverse in its cause of diseases than just being associated with high blood cholesterol, high blood pressure and obesity. Syndrome X, with its characteristic component of insulin resistance, can contribute to infertility, irregular menstruation, polycystic ovary syndrome (PCOS), fatty liver, inflammation in the body and the development of certain types of cancer.

Expanding our knowledge of the problems associated with Syndrome X led to my desire to rename Syndrome X as Syndrome X, Y and Z… (Holt S, "Combat Syndrome X, Y and Z…," Wellness Publishing, Newark, NJ, 2002). Syndrome X is caused by poor lifestyle, excess simple sugar in the diet, lack of exercise, and hereditary tendencies. When I discuss the factors that have tipped the balance towards obesity in Western society, I am also addressing the constellation of obesity-related disorders that must not be divorced from considerations of weight problems or obesity alone. My reiterations are justified.

Hereditary Factors Contribute to Weight Gain

While hereditary tendencies appear to operate in the obesity epidemic, it is still important to realize that genes of the body (hereditary material) interact with the environment. Our genetic tendencies are shaped by our environment. The presence of certain genetic material in some people does not mean that obesity or Syndrome X is an inevitable occurrence. It occurs because the susceptible person is more sensitive to the lifestyle choices that "tip the balance" towards being overweight, with or without the presence of Syndrome X. Without the imposition of the "Syndrome X-forming lifestyle" on the susceptible person, Syndrome X may not be an inevitable occurrence.

My notions about a lack of necessity for the development of obesity, Syndrome X or maturity onset diabetes mellitus are supported by science. Careful population studies in two groups of Pima Indians living either in Arizona or Northern Mexico, show great differences in obesity rates, cardiovascular risk factors and heart health. The combination of problems in Syndrome X and maturity onset diabetes are rife among the Pima in Arizona, but they are quite uncommon in the Pima from Northern Mexico. This difference is clearly associated with differences in lifestyle, where the Pima in Arizona has embraced the modern American "way of life," but the Mexican Pima still farms, remains active and remains a "relative" stranger to the "American lifestyle."

Diseases of Plentitude

The modern "conveniences" of what we believe to be "advanced" lifestyles are tipping the balance, such that our metabolic evolution has accelerated in the wrong direction in recent times. Our metabolic evolution has moved rapidly towards a status of the metabolic Syndrome X (weight gain, hypercholesterolemia and hypertension, linked by insulin resistance). Along with Syndrome X come other diseases to provide a "new-found" unifying concept of chronic degenerative disease (Syndrome X, Y and Z...).

One must reflect upon whether the solution to this problem rests in conventional drug treatments or "magic bullet" medicine. The solution to lifestyle problems rests in the correction of lifestyle, and the notion of a "lifestyle drug" for the treatment of obesity or Syndrome X may be quite preposterous. That said, drugs to treat Syndrome X are becoming the "apple of the pharmaceutical industries' eyes."

An Unfitness Revolution?

Physical activity experts in the 1980s could not have predicted today's "gloomy" statistics on the health of the nation. Surveys in the 1980's revealed the start of the modern-day, acceleration in the occurrences of weight gain, Syndrome X and maturity onset diabetes mellitus. These findings are notable in young people, and they have been highlighted in studies published recently (e.g. Ford ES, Giles WH and Dietz WH, Prevalence of the Metabolic Syndrome (*Syndrome X*) Among US Adults, JAMA 287, 3, 356-359, 2002).

The public health observations of the 1970s and 1980s showed children to be "in poor shape," compared with their counterparts, a decade or so earlier. These observations heralded prophecies of endangered health of the nation. While the message of "endangerment" of the nation continues to be communicated, little has happened in public health initiatives to reverse trends for an "overweight America." The message of "endangerment" has been replaced in recent times by more of an acute public health emergency, with the revelation of the "obesity pandemic."

The Theory of Excess

There is no shortage of recreational possibilities, gymnasia or playgrounds in the US, but we have the most idle kids in the world and the U.S. has among the highest rates of occurrence of degenerative disease. Modern-day health problems in the US are not examples of deficiency diseases; they fall more into "the disease theory of excess."

The excesses in Western societies include, but are not limited to, excessive calories, delicious abundant junk food, the idle, entertainment of TVs, VCRs and computers, etc. Many Americans drive everywhere and snack on junk food, while they engage in passive entertainment. American healthcare is the most advanced in the world, but it is not portable to the economically disadvantaged. U.S. healthcare is focused on disease diagnosis and management, not on preventive medicine. What many Americans have perceived as improvements in lifestyle are often the antithesis of activity that will promote health and well-being.

Chapter Summary

Weight gain, the metabolic Syndrome X, pre-diabetes and the development of maturity onset (Type 2) diabetes mellitus are inextricably linked. These are best viewed as lifestyle disorders, typified by a combined lack of physical activity, poor nutrition and hereditary tendencies. Our "advanced" lifestyle has created a major, modern challenge to health and well-being.

Simple sugars in the diet have been implicated as a key cause of the "weight problem", facing many people. However, this is not the whole story. Low carb diets became an attractive option for weight control, but such diets are not a complete approach when used alone (vide infra).

The information on obesity related illness, reviewed in this chapter, sets the stage for Hoodia gordonii as a potential factor among Syndrome X Nutritional Factors®. These factors are natural supplements that are useful in the combat against Syndrome X (www.combatsyndromex.com).

CHAPTER 4

A HEALTHY WEIGHT CONTROL INITIATIVE

Diet Guidelines

Many people can shed a few pounds in the short term, but few obese individuals achieve or maintain their weight loss targets.

I can start to define dietary principles and recommendations for macronutrient intakes in terms of calories and ratios of inclusion (the amount and type of fat, carbohydrates and protein in the diet) to combat obesity and Syndrome X. The general principles that are applied in a diet to combat obesity and Syndrome X involve:

- A reduction of carbohydrate intake in the form of simple sugars. Up to 40% of the diet can come from carbohydrates preferably of the complex type. Induction phases in low carb diets with more stringent carbohydrate restriction are not harmful, if undertaken only for a couple of weeks or so.

- Eating foods with a low Glycemic Index. Foods that cause high swings in blood glucose and promote insulin secretion make Syndrome X worse. Substitution of complex carbohydrates and fiber are recommended.

- Intakes of "healthy types of fats" can be more liberal than proposed in nationally acclaimed diets, e.g. USDA Food Pyramid or American Heart Association recommendations. An effective diet to combat Syndrome X may derive 40% of its calories from fat, but this fat must be of a healthy type, especially Omega-3 fatty acids, or fish oil.

- Only about 10%-15% of the diet needs to come from protein. Excessive protein intake especially of meat or dairy origin is linked to many chronic degenerative diseases and components of protein (certain amino acids) can cause insulin release, at least by promoting gluconeogenesis (sugar formation from protein). More liberal vegetable protein intake is advisable.

- Calories should not be reduced below about 1400 calories per day, without medical supervision.

I reiterate my belief that all fixed dietary recommendations possess disadvantages or limitations; and I stress the frequent need to obtain expert nutritional advice to tailor a diet to an individual's needs.

Out of a lack of consensus about diets, I believe that certain issues become clear:

1. Calorie control in the diet is mandatory and any diet cannot work without exercise, behavior modification and change from adverse to positive lifestyle

2. Cutting back on dietary saturated fats and cholesterol (the foundation of the AHA diet) is beneficial. This clear fact disqualifies some aspects of the original Atkins' Diet from being heart-healthy. In recent times, the value of healthy fats of the omega 3 series has been recognized. The AHA will not "come clean" on the negative consequences of refined carbohydrates, because of their stubborn support of the U.S. Food Guide Pyramid.

3. Excessive animal protein intake does not, itself, cause weight loss; it is associated with chronic disease (e.g. osteoporosis) and it often comes along with saturated fat. These issues tend to question aspects of the Atkins' or the Zone Diet. Furthermore, proteins can be broken down into amino acids that will promote insulin secretion. Excessive animal protein is best avoided in weight control diets and Syndrome X management, but the same may not be true of vegetable protein, e.g. soy protein.

4. The type of fat in the diet is much more important than previously recognized. Mono and polyunsaturated fats (oils) that are not adulterated (hydrogenated to form trans-fatty acids) are generally healthy. However, the omega 6 to omega 3 unsaturated fatty acid balance is very important. It should be as close to 1:1 as possible.

5. Diets to curb insulin resistance must limit simple sugars, saturated fats and salt, but may contain more liberal amounts of "healthy fat", with careful concern for their calorie content, to avoid weight gain. Protein metabolism in the presence of glucose intolerance is often disturbed and excessive animal protein intake may be undesirable.

6. The "Glycemic Index" of food is an important principle that is simple to understand and apply without the need for laborious calculations of the Glycemic Index of various foods. This index measures the ability of any given food to shoot up levels of blood glucose and insulin.

7. Selected dietary supplements and functional foods are of value in the "first-line attack" against the components of Syndrome X, e.g. dietary fiber, beta glucan fractions of soluble oat fiber, soy protein, chromium, alpha lipoic acid, antioxidants and omega 3 fatty acids (e.g. Syndrome X Nutritional Factors, www.naturesbenefit.com).

8. Hoodia gordonii may be a major factor in controlling calorie intakes in the diet.

Overall, my dietary recommendations to combat obesity and/or Syndrome X do not exist as "stand-alone" interventions. Leading healthcare organizations and many researchers stress that weight control programs must incorporate lifestyle, behavior change and perhaps other natural options. (intentional echolalia!)

More Fruit and Vegetables

The fruit-vegetable and grain groups are highly desirable components of a diet for cardiovascular health. The only limitation to this aspect of the diet is to watch total calorie intake. An individual with a "big appetite" (a high satiety level) is advised to fill up with vegetables that have a low calorie density (and a low glycemic index). The concept of caloric density of food is important. Certain foods are more "dilute" in calories than others because of their variable composition of protein, fat, carbohydrate and fiber.

Dietary Sugars

It would be wrong to continue to talk about restriction of simple sugars in the diet without defining these items in detail. There are several simple sugars which occur commonly in foods. These sugars are found in both processed and natural foods. Glucose is a simple sugar that can appear in the bloodstream, as a result of eating other simple sugars, such as sucrose (table sugar). Sugar tastes good to most people, especially children.

Table 2 lists a variety of simple sugars that occur in the diet. This table is useful in the overall identification of foods that are to be avoided in the "modified low carb diet" that I have proposed for weight control.

Sugar	Sources
Sucrose	Otherwise called common table sugar. Sucrose is added as a sweetener to many foods e.g. cookies, desserts, etc. Sucrose is a disaccharide made up of glucose and fructose.
Fructose	Fructose is a popular cheap sweetener used in many foods, especially carbonated soda. It is found in many fruits and honey. While it is handled by the body in a different way than glucose, it is still a miscreant in the cause of weight gain, etc.
Glucose	Glucose is found in fruits and it is often added to foods as a sweetener. It enters the body directly into the bloodstream and it is what one refers to as "blood sugar."

Maltose

This sugar is found in several vegetables and it is a key ingredient of sprouted seeds and malted beverages, e.g. beer. Maltose is often added to processed foods and it is derived from the breakdown of starches.

Lactose

Lactose is found in milk and several dairy products. Intolerance to lactose in the diet causes general gastrointestinal upset (lactose intolerance). Lactose is a disaccharide made up of glucose and galactose.

Table 2: Simple sugars in the diet

Eureka? A Fight Against Obesity and Syndrome X?

The solution to making the obesity or weight gain problem go away, while reducing the occurrence of its associated diseases, is for many people a combat against insulin resistance and compensatory increases in blood insulin. This insulin resistance is the absolute hallmark of the metabolic Syndrome X that affects at least one in four of the U.S. population.

The dietary temptations of day-to-day living in Western society are so great that any "fixed diet" cannot be applied in continuity. The result is that weight control does not occur in continuity. However, an intervention that may make the difference is the use of lifestyle changes and dietary supplements consisting of measured amounts of the correct foods, food extracts and nutrients that can help to reverse insulin resistance and the associated excess secretion of insulin by the body. Calorie control is a key issue; and the appetite suppressing properties of Hoodia gordonii would be a great help in controlling Syndrome X (www.hoodiasupreme.com)

These concepts of blunting blood sugar and blood insulin responses are at the basis of the development of the formulas of dietary supplements, such as LowCarb Diet Facilitator™ and Syndrome X Nutritional Factors™ (www.naturesbenefit.com). I believe that low, refined-carbohydrate "lifestyles" are indisputably beneficial, but they require facilitation. Dietary supplements can be adjuncts to make low carb dietary approaches more effective in many ways (www.naturesbenefit.com).

For a "low carbohydrate diet" to work, a combat against insulin resistance must often be facilitated.

Farmyard Science

Understanding a rational approach to diet in modern times requires an acknowledgment of how we became overweight. In a simplistic manner, an understanding of weight gain can begin in the farmyard. The farmer fattens hens or other domestic animals by a combination of restraint (lack of exercise) and the feeding of excess calories in the animals' diet. If the farmer has "economics" in mind, the cheapest source of calories will be used to fatten the animal. Welcome to America!

This situation is readily comparable with the evolution of the "Standard American Diet" (SAD), which is underpinned by the "fast or junk food industries." By adding a sedentary lifestyle, Americans may have reproduced the farmers' tactics on how to effectively fatten the animal. Eating cheap, "fast" or processed food and lounging around are common among Americans and other "Westerners." Figure 2 shows our weight gain linked to the new epidemic of Type II diabetes mellitus. This is "diabesity".

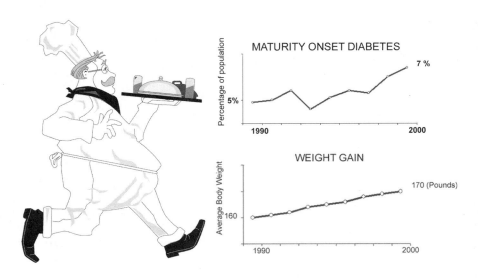

Figure 2: As the nation's weight rises, the occurrence of maturity onset diabetes mellitus gallops. Notice the short period (10 years) in which this tragic situation has emerged. This illustration supports Atkins' notion of "diabesity."

Chapter Summary

While the adoption of a modified low carb diet is a step in the right direction, many scientific observations point to the limitations of diets alone for weight control. Simple sugars in the diet trigger Syndrome X and weight gain, but many other factors operate. The careful modification of low carb diets with added lifestyle strategies and other nutritional interventions can make a "low carb diet approach" more effective for weight control and healthier overall. Weight control must occur with a focus on general health, and controlling calorie intake in the diet is recognized as a key factor in weight loss. This notion reinforces our interest in the dictary, calorie control that may be achieved with Hoodia gordonii.

CHAPTER 5

ADVICE BEYOND DIETS

Lifestyle, Obesity, and Syndrome X

Researchers have started to show how genetic tendencies and body form (fatness, aerobic fitness levels, etc.) alter the ability of an individual to handle sugar in the diet (glucose tolerance). Studies in families show the occurrence of insulin resistance among relatives. This finding confirms the importance of hereditary tendencies towards obesity and Syndrome X, but genetics do not explain the whole picture.

Many studies have shown how adverse lifestyle can increase cardiovascular risk and contribute variably to the initiation and progression of weight gain and Syndrome X. The cardinal components of Syndrome X are risks for cardiovascular disease. Physical activity improves the handling of sugar by the body and works against insulin resistance. Smoking enhances resistance to insulin, as does excessive alcohol drinking and excessive intake of caffeine (cola and coffee). Poor diet with excessive consumption of calories and refined carbohydrates is a prime cause of obesity, Syndrome X and ultimately Type 2 diabetes.

Foods that do not cause rapid rises in blood sugar – low glycemic foods — are valuable in the combat against insulin resistance, hyperinsulinemia, Syndrome X and Type 2 diabetes. Excessive intake of salt, saturated fat, and protein of animal origin contributes to the progression of Syndrome X. Being fat (obesity) is particularly damaging to health, largely because insulin resistance and obesity go "hand in hand."

Smoothing-Out Blood Glucose Levels

It is clear that a poor diet containing excess refined sugar and unhealthy types of fat plays a major role in causing insulin resistance and the evolution of Syndrome X, obesity, pre-diabetes and Type 2 diabetes mellitus. Simple sugars are consumed in Western society in staggering amounts. These sugars "gyrate" blood sugar and test the insulin controls in the body. Sugar is the prime stimulus to cause insulin secretion. Unfortunately, sugar comes with many positive behavioral reinforcements. It tastes good and satisfies the cravings which are caused by insulin resistance itself! This is a "vicious cycle" of events.

Refined sugar may be recognized by the individual as alleviating temporarily symptoms of "food craving" associated with Syndrome X and an overweight body status. These circumstances apply especially if intermittent hypoglycemia (low blood sugar) occurs. Intermittent low blood sugar causes intermittent craving for sugar in people with obesity, Syndrome X and diabetes. This is a vicious cycle that must be broken. Smoothing out blood glucose or sensitizing the actions of insulin with dietary supplements can help to break this vicious cycle.

The promotion of insulin secretion in the presence of insulin resistance will tend to make obesity and Syndrome X "gallop" in this progression. (www.combatsyndromex.com).

Behavior Modification and Guidelines for Weight Control

I stress that successful weight control can only occur by modifications of poor day- to-day habits, especially eating behavior. Many individuals have developed eating habits that work against efforts to control calorie intake and promote exercise. Several specific suggestions can be made on behavior modification, as part of a weight control plan:

- **Recognize calorie contents of various foods and establish a target for calorie intake. It is necessary to review on a regular basis whether or not calorie intake goals have been met.**
- **Choose low calorie, low glycemic index foods, and if snacking is planned then healthy, reduced-caloric snacks must be used.**
- **Avoid "temptations" or external influences that precipitate eating. Plan what you want to eat rather than selecting from set menus and prepare only as much food as meets the calorie goals that have been set.**
- **Think about calories not about food and treat yourself for meeting the calorie intake. Do not use food as a reward.**
- **Heighten your awareness of body feelings that make you eat. Do not eat past hunger signals. Pause during a meal and ask**

yourself if your appetite is satisfied.
- Use your imagination creatively. Imagine that you feel lousy after overeating – remember the feeling. Look in a mirror when you want to binge or imagine that you have just eaten.
- Do not take two steps forward and three back. Accept occasional failures and never permit them to be an excuse to give up.
- Solve the problem with a greater awareness of your ability to reason. Do not succumb to victimizing statements about weight.
- Every failure must be a lesson learned. Educate yourself about nutrition and lifestyle or review what you already know.
- Work on avoiding the "sweet tooth."
- Do not set unrealistic weight loss goals.

Exercise

Exercise can make important contributions to all aspects of physical and mental well-being. If there was a true "health panacea," one may choose exercise as the first-line option. Before commencing an exercise program, it is important that the individual check with his or her physician or professional trainer. A physician should be able to give some advice about the type and amount of exercise that is ideal, but certified professional trainers or physiotherapists are often more knowledgeable about exercise tolerance and the matching of different types of exercise to physical or health needs.

There are some misconceptions about the role of exercise in lifestyle. An individual may set an expectation that is too great, and it is known that an individual's ability to undertake an exercise depends on his or her physical condition, age and general health. Unlike sportsmen or women who need to train very arduously, most individuals should not push exercise to the limits.

Exercise and Global Well-Being

Physical exercise becomes increasingly important for health, especially as the nation ages. Unfortunately, the odds are sometimes stacked against the engagement of exercise by mature people. However, the good news is that health can come from modest daily exercise. Medical experts usually advise that people over the age of 50 years should have at least 30 minutes of exercise per day; and even gentle exercise is health-giving (e.g. walking, simple household chores, etc.).

Exercise may be best undertaken in a gymnasium where supervision can occur. However, all kinds of exercise are healthful, including walking, cycling, swimming or tending to jobs around the home. It is useful for individuals to understand the basic kinds of exercise and their relative benefits, but all forms of exercise can help to maintain well-being (Table 3).

TYPES OF EXERCISE AND THEIR BENEFITS

Type	Specific Benefits	Examples
Flexibility (stretch) Exercises	Increases range of movement and helps prepare for strenuous exercise	Stretch routines
Endurance Training	Improves heart and breathing functions; Prevents Syndrome X and maturity onset diabetes mellitus; May prevent stroke, heart attack and some types of cancer.	Walking, running, swimming, cycling
Strength Training	Builds muscles and benefits body metabolism; Affords good control of blood sugar useful for weight control; Very important to combat Syndrome X; Prevents thin bones (osteoporosis)	Weight training, bowflex training, resistance machines
Balance Exercises	A major part of injury prevention and very important in the elderly where osteoporosis and injuries spell trouble	Extension of the limbs with balance
Special Exercises	Yoga and Tai-chi	Many health benefits

Table 3: Types of exercise and their potential benefits.

Many Beneficial Outcomes of Exercise

Exercise has a direct beneficial effect on the heart, lungs, muscles, joints and bones. It is a very important adjunct to diet in a weight loss program where calories need to be expended and fat accumulation may diminish. Exercise is an important aid to rehabilitation following any illness. If exercise is sustained for at least 15 minutes on a daily basis, it results in improvements in cardiovascular and respiratory functions of the body. In addition, exercise helps to combat insulin resistance, lower blood sugar; and it prevents diabetes mellitus and Syndrome X.

Routine daily exercise and workouts have a preventative benefit in terms of respiratory and circulatory diseases. Exercise increases circulation and improves muscle tone and strength. It is possible to benefit from exercise in many different forms, including walking, housework, jogging, biking, swimming or doing a series of stretching exercises.

Regular exercise, even if it is not strenuous, will help burn calories and play an important adjunctive role in dieting and the management of obesity. Thus, exercise is a great helper in weight control and the combat against Syndrome X. There is a common misconception that a "workout" has to be very strenuous in order to burn calories. This is not necessarily the case, especially for the reformed "couch potato."

A Contrarian Thought: Stress and Weight Gain

One could reach some contrarian opinions about weight control, while reflecting on the role of stress in causing obesity. It is right to assume that periods of relaxation, interspersed with exercise may be very important in controlling weight gain – a factor not "stressed" in obesity management. In other words, sitting and worrying about not going to the gymnasium may be more dangerous than skipping the odd visit!

There are clear biochemical explanations why stress causes obesity, weight gain and Syndrome X. When the stress hormone cortisol is released, it releases sugar and fatty acids into the bloodstream. Blood sugar rises stimulate insulin production and cause secondary rises in blood pressure and blood cholesterol. Being somewhat "laid back" mentally is clearly an advantage for heart health and these observations reinforce the idea of controlling the stress-producing Type A behavior that creeps into many American lives. Type A ("hyper"-behavior) is a risk for heart attack.

The Glycemic Index: A Concept to Embrace

The "Glycemic Index" is a way of describing the ability of different foods to cause a rise in blood sugar. Foods laden with simple sugars can be expected to cause a rapid rise in blood glucose. These sugary foods are the prime examples of foods with a "high Glycemic Index." It is possible to rank foods within the context of the Glycemic Index. In fact, foods can be given a Glycemic Index Score by comparing their effects on blood glucose in comparison to a reference food, such as pure glucose or white bread.

The Glycemic Index has been described as a groundbreaking medical discovery that should guide dietary choices for wellness promotion. While the Glycemic Index is a useful concept, it is not a new discovery. Its role in planning diets for weight loss and health promotion has been emphasized in a dozen recent books, but the concepts may have been "hyped" in their application.

I propose that the concept of the Glycemic Index can be interpreted, in major part, in terms of simple gastrointestinal physiology. The factors that control the rate at which sugars are absorbed from food were well documented prior to the description of the "Glycemic Index." Changes in the rate at which the stomach empties food to its principal site of digestion in the small intestine underlies the concept of the Glycemic Index (Holt S. et al, Lancet, 1, 636-9, 1979). Let me explain.

Glycemic Index and Load: Useful Guidelines

The Glycemic Index or glycemic load of foods gives people a useful guideline to identify foods that are best avoided to prevent or manage excessive weight and Syndrome X. The major problem of scoring foods with a numerical Glycemic Index is that these indices are calculated from the act of eating one food at a time. In a normal diet, few people eat one item alone. Table 4 gives a partial list of common foods and their "guesstimated" glycemic indices.

GLYCEMIC INDEX VALUES

High	Intermediate	Low
>74	>51 to <74	<50
White bread	Whole wheat bread	Oatmeal
Sugar-laden breakfast cereals	Cereals with less sugar	Milk, dairy
Potatoes	Sports nutrition bars	Soy foods
Candies	"Sweet" fruits	"Less sweet" fruits
Many "fat-free" foods	Fiber-containing bagels	Beans

Table 4: The above Glycemic Index chart is a truncated version of the painstaking calculation of glycemic indices of foods. Foods containing simple sugars can be classified on a scale of 1 to 100 in the jargon of the Glycemic Index pundits. The scale is the speed at which sugar enters the bloodstream, i.e. the RATE. This is a major function of the rate at which the stomach empties the food. Many factors affect the rate at which the stomach empties (Holt S, Gastric Emptying: Control and Management. Survey of Digestive Diseases 3, 4:210-229, 1985). Glycemic indices and glycemic loads can vary in the same category of foods, e.g., white flour bagels can be of high Glycemic Index whereas plain bagels with much fiber can cross over to levels of an intermediate or even low Glycemic Index.

Blunting the Blood Glucose and Insulin Response

The principal cause of rapid high swings in blood glucose and secondarily blood insulin is the intake of refined carbohydrates, usually in the form of sucrose (table sugar). Sucrose is a combination of two small sugars (monosaccharides fructose and glucose). Fructose is increasingly used as a sweetener in food and beverages because it is cheap to produce on a commercial basis. While fructose is handled by the body somewhat differently from glucose, fructose is still a "miscreant" when it comes to unwanted upward swings in blood glucose and blood insulin, especially in the presence of insulin resistance.

Figure 3 shows how blood glucose can rise rapidly to high levels following the intake of simple sugars. Within Figure 3 is an example of the use of soluble fiber (guar gum, pectin or oat soluble fiber) to blunt rises in blood glucose. In Figure 3 one can see how blunting the glucose response will similarly blunt the insulin response. This effect is attributable to the ability of sticky, soluble fiber to delay the rate at which the stomach empties (Holt et al., 1979).

Glucose and other substances are mainly absorbed in the small intestine, beyond the stomach. The greater the rate at which the stomach empties its contents increases the rate at which nutrients, such as glucose, are presented to their site of maximal absorption in the small intestine. Thus, the more rapid the stomach-emptying, the quicker glucose moves into the intestine where it rapidly enters the bloodstream. Rapid glucose entry into the bloodstream causes high blood sugars which drive the pancreas to secrete insulin.

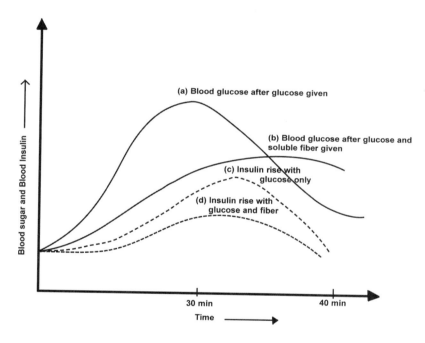

Figure 3: "Blunting" of blood glucose and insulin responses following a meal or the ingestion of glucose. Derived in part from data presented by Holt S. et al, Lancet, 1, 636-9, 1979 and reproduced in a "diagrammatic" form. When soluble fiber is taken with glucose the blood glucose curve over time is "flattened" to a major degree. This "blunts" the rise in blood glucose and, secondarily, the rise in insulin levels after fiber is taken. These observations explain the Glycemic Index of foods, to a major degree, in single meals.

Sleep, Obesity, and Syndrome X

Sleep deprivation causes resistance to the actions of the hormone insulin, even in healthy people. Given insulin's role in weight control, blood pressure and blood cholesterol regulation, one can see how changes in insulin's action, in the "wrong direction," may favor the development of common diseases, such as cardiovascular disease. It has been defined that high levels of insulin, in the presence of resistance to the actions of the hormone insulin on blood glucose, may lead to heart disease, diabetes and cancer (Holt S, "Combat Syndrome X, Y and Z....," Wellness Publishing, Newark, NJ, 2002).

The modern epidemic of Syndrome X is linked to sleeplessness which is linked to other factors such as stress. Recent studies in more than 4,000 schoolchildren have linked stress with obesity. While stress may tend to cause children to eat more, it also causes sleep deprivation. The researchers in these recent studies of stress and obesity in children have tended to focus their conclusions on calorie intake. However, I believe that the modern epidemic of sleep deprivation plays a major role in weight gain and obesity. The whole situation is a vicious cycle because stress aggravates the components of Syndrome X and contributes to their ability to damage health (www.sleepnaturally.com).

Chapter Summary

In Syndrome X, insulin resistance leads to excess circulating blood insulin. Abnormalities in the ability of the body to handle sugar in the diet result in glucose intolerance. Added to this is the evolution of obesity, high blood cholesterol and high blood pressure. Many diseases are caused by this complex change in body metabolism. A nutritional approach with lifestyle intervention is the key to reversing the abnormalities of body chemistry in the overweight individual or the person with Syndrome X. Blunting the rapid swings of blood glucose and insulin with soluble fiber is a key approach in the combat against Syndrome X and obesity.

CHAPTER 6

THE SCIENCE OF HOODIA (ANIMALS)

Weight Control is Back to Basics

So far in this book, I trust that readers have dispelled the myth that a "magic diet" exists on the horizon. It is known that weight control is a function of many factors, other than diet alone. I must reiterate that there cannot be sustained weight loss without modification of behavior, control of calorie intake, exercise for energy expenditure, and a healthy lifestyle. Obesity is rapidly becoming the number one preventable cause of death in many western societies. In fact, even in industrialized areas of third-world countries, emerging affluence and over-nutrition has created an epidemic of obesity and Type II diabetes mellitus. This is the issue of "diabesity". Controlling the amount of food eaten and type of food eaten are very important in the new healthy weight control initiative. Controlling the amount of food eaten may be modified by behavior change, with the help of Hoodia gordonii.

Studies of individuals who have managed to engage in sustained weight control show that these successful people used much more than diet alone to control weight in the long term. A key factor in successful long-term weight control is behavior modification. The idea of behavior modification for weight control has been bandied around for many years, but the bottom line means taking control of our "social gluttony." In other words, learning to select appropriate meal portion sizes and control calorie intake, by psychological or social maneuvers, are germane for the control of the nation's waistline.

Heralding Hoodia?

I wish to go beyond the usual advice about diet and I take a focus on how the body regulates hunger, appetite, and satiety. I believe that lack of control of appetite, together with an increasing learned-ability to eat beyond the satiety signals, causes over indulgence. These are key factors in fueling the obesity epidemic in Western society. We have entered the realm of a whole host of diseases linked to obesity and caused by plentitude. Modern humankind will not subscribe to the known dangers of "the theory of excess." However, modern science has provided a new hope in facilitating the modification of behavior that causes overeating. This modern science draws upon the folklore history of the San bushmen of South Africa, who unraveled the secret of Hoodia gordonii. Hoodia gordonii is heralded as a modern weight loss miracle, and the science behind the hope of Hoodia must be examined.

Scientists and desperate people afflicted by excessive weight gain or obesity are appropriately excited about the possibility of the maintenance of a healthy weight. It stands to reason that people who are overweight would be attracted to a way of controlling weight that could be somewhat passive, if Hoodia fulfills its promise of taking away appetite. I believe that the promise of Hoodia is very real. A person who is not hungry after they take Hoodia will be less likely to overindulge and "put on pounds". The mechanism by which Hoodia gordonii accomplishes appetite, hunger, or thirst suppression is becoming increasingly understood from basic science experiments and clinical observations.

How Does Hoodia gordonii Work?

Hoodia gordonii appears to contain special components (molecules) that act upon specific regions of the brain to promote a feeling of fullness. In this regard, Hoodia gordonii has an ability to "play a trick" on the brain, by giving the central nervous system a powerful message that a person is full (satiated). This feeling of fullness occurs because Hoodia gives a satiety signal to the hypothalamus, a small area of the underside of the brain.

As previously discussed, tribesman in arid regions of the South African desert have used species of Hoodia for appetite and thirst suppression. It is stated that the earliest observation of the use of Hoodia by the bushmen was made in the 1930's, but in the 1960's San bushmen reported the traditional use of Hoodia to members of the South African Army. This information on the folklore use of Hoodia was acted upon in the 1960's by the Council for Scientific and Industrial Research (CSIR) of South Africa. This research agency performed animal studies that showed striking reduction in food intake and weight loss when

Hoodia was added to the diet of rats.

These observations with Hoodia administration to animals were believed to be due to the suppression of hunger and appetite, because no toxicity occurred in animals, that could be ascribed to the use of Hoodia. The findings were so enlightening that the CSIR filed several patents on components of Hoodia species (Hoodia gordonii and Hoodia lugardi) and other species of a family of plants called Trichocaulon.

After testing many concentrates of the plant Hoodia gordonii, researchers concluded that the biological activity for appetite suppression in Hoodia was centered around its content of steroidal glycoside molecules. It has been proposed in several patents that these bioactive components of Hoodia could be used for appetite suppression, weight loss, and the management of the metabolic Syndrome X. The potential value of Hoodia in the management of metabolic Syndrome X rests upon the idea that weight management will alter insulin resistance and the presence of coexisting cardiovascular risk factors, such as high blood cholesterol, or high blood pressure.

Biological Activity in Experimental Animals

The effect of Hoodia on food intake was studied in "poor" rats. In the early experiments, reported in 2001, the effect of the Hoodia plant on food intake and body weight was studied in rats who were either lean or obese, based on their own genetic pre-dispositions. These experiments showed that the animals who received Hoodia had rapid onset of decreased food intake, which was sustained over a period of weeks. This resulted in major degrees of weight loss in the rats. The researchers repeated these early experiments and used a crude concentration of dried Hoodia gordonii in "free-feeding" rats. Again, they found marked and continuous reductions in food intake. It is understood that rats will eat almost anything, and they will gorge themselves to a degree of excess. Knocking out the appetite or hunger drive of a rat is a dramatic event!

Attention was focused on the Hoodia-treated "fat rats" which lost almost twice the amount of body weight compared with "thin rats". Careful measurements were made of fat distribution in these experimental animals. It was found that body fat in certain areas was reduced by a factor of 50% in obese rats, compared to similar animals on a conventional diet that did not include Hoodia. Even the thin rats reduced their body weight by a factor of one fifth.

The rats appeared to remain healthy despite their weight loss, and in separate experiments large does of Hoodia have been given to rats to see if any toxic reactions occur. It appears that even large doses of Hoodia have no ill effects on "dear" rats. I lament the use of animals in scientific research, but we can thank these rats for showing us that they shared the effect of Hoodia on appetite suppression with humans.

There have been many anecdotal reports from native South Africans and from hundreds of people in Western society that confirm that Hoodia gordonii can diminish sensations of hunger or thirst. It should be noted that the dramatic effect of Hoodia on appetite suppression has been experienced with the whole plant or crude extract. The precedent for safety of the use of Hoodia in the food chain is in this "whole" form. For these reasons scientists in the dietary supplement industry have become excited about the real possibility of an all-natural dietary supplement product that could assist in behavior modification for weight control, by taking the edge off appetite (www.hoodiasupreme.com).

Patent Rights?

The rights to patents on components of the Hoodia plant (steroidal glycosides) have been transferred for commercialization through a corporation in Cambridge England called Phytopharm, PLC. In a chain of events to commercialize the use of Hoodia, patents have been assessed and or potentially acquired by the pharmaceutical industry. At the time of writing, the food giant Unilever Inc. reported that it had gained the exclusive worldwide rights to an appetite-suppressing compound extracted from the Hoodia gordonii plant by Phytopharm PLC in England. It has been estimated that these new Hoodia extracts, placed into food products, may reach the market in the year 2008 or thereabouts. The highly effective and popular product, Slim-Fast, seems to be a potential target for the addition of Hoodia in the future. Unilever has estimated that this product could be used by almost one billion people worldwide who are "fighting the flab."

Hard Science in Experimental Animals

In an important article published in the scientific journal "Brain Research", in April 2004, researchers from Brown Medical School in

Providence, RI (US) described elegant animal experiments that show the effects of components of Hoodia on the central nervous system. These authors reflected on earlier research in the "poor" fat and thin rats. They expanded earlier observations by describing beneficial effects of Hoodia extracts (concentrates containing many components) on rats who are born to be fat and diabetic (Zucker Rats).

These "fat rats" are bred to be obese and they are called "Zucker rats". In these rats with "diabesity" (diabetes and obesity), Hoodia suppressed appetite and assisted in the reversal of diabetes, as long as the rats ate the Hoodia. These fat, diabetic rats lost weight even though they were fed an abundant, delicious diet (delicious for a rat). It was stated again, in this scientific article, that animal safety studies did not show bad side effects on the experimental animals, even though accelerated weight loss occurred. Recently, there have been studies in small groups of humans which have shown that there are no apparent toxic effects of taking concentrated forms of Hoodia. In addition, up to thousands of people have taken Hoodia gordonii in dietary supplements without any known, significant, adverse effects.

Steroidal Glycosides

Researchers have focused their attention on particular compounds (steroidal glycosides) as the active appetite-suppressant constituents of Hoodia. These steroidal glycosides are similar to a group of compounds that are sometimes called "cardenolides". This group of natural, chemical compounds are "glycosides" and many of these compounds often work on pumping mechanisms that control the sodium or potassium content of cells. However, it would appear that the steroidal glycosides in Hoodia may not work primarily by altering these energy dependent "pumps" that occur in cells of the body. Many people think that glycosides are compounds that are mainly active on the heart, e.g., digitalis or digoxin, but the glycosides in Hoodia appear different; and they do not affect the heart to any demonstrable degree.

Complex Animal Experiments

The studies on how components of Hoodia may work to suppress appetite in animals involved complex laboratory procedures. In brief, fractions of Hoodia enriched with steroidal glycosides were given to laboratory rats who were treated well with adequate food and water intake, in most circumstances of the experiments.

Extracts of Hoodia were given by injection into the head of the rat and into the rat's brain. The rats were then killed humanely, and various estimations of the chemistry of various parts of the brain were measured. In some cases, measurements were made in cultures of cells taken from specific areas of rats' brains, such as the hypothalamus.

A variety of complicated measurements were made under various conditions of experiments, and significant effects were noted. In simplistic terms, the experiments in rats showed that Hoodia extracts could increase energy content in the nerve cells of the hypothalamus of the brain. This is an area of the brain that is involved in hunger, appetite, satiety, blood pressure, hormonal and temperature regulation. The hypothalamus is an area of the brain that takes multiple messages and gives multiple signals for a variety of body functions.

The rat studies performed by these researchers led to their conclusion that an important mechanism of the regulation of food intake by the hypothalamus of the brain is the alteration of the hypothalamic cells' contents of energy in the form of ATP (adenosine triphosphate, a principle energy-containing compound of the body). This conclusion requires further validation; and I would question that this is the whole explanation of mechanism of the regulation of food intake that is noted with Hoodia. I would further question that this is the only mechanism of effect of Hoodia material extracts on other body functions.

Increases in Energy in the Hypothalamus

The researchers were looking mainly to find out "just how" the steroidal glycoside molecules caused their appetite-suppressant effect. It should be noted that the researchers disclosed that dried whole plant ,as well as purified extract have been noted in many previous studies to cause appetite suppression when given by mouth, or injection. The main finding in these important animal experiment was that the steroidal glycosides in Hoodia resulted in increases in measured, energy content in nerve cells in the brain (ATP) by a factor of 50 to 150%. This occurred specifically in the nerve cells in the hypothalamus of rats.

Injecting Hoodia extracts into more remote areas of the brain (third ventricle) showed alterations in energy content in the hypothalamus. This demonstrates the importance of interconnecting areas of the brain that are involved in sensing the body's intake of energy (food). Thus, the hypothalamus seems to be the "switch box" or "integrator" of appetite and it accepts signals from the body and other parts of the brain.

The Complex Nature of Energy Regulation

Elegant biochemical, molecular and genetic studies continue to contribute to an overall understanding of the regulation of energy balance, hunger, appetite and satiety, by the brain and other body organs. While many different messenger molecules (neurotransmitters and hormones), involved in energy control in the body, have been discovered, the precise interaction of many of these pathways of signals that regulate feeding behavior, or sensations that control food intake, remains unknown. It is appreciated that satiety signals involve many body functions such as digestive function (e.g., gastric emptying), and smell and taste (olfactory) senses. Furthermore, nutrient concentrations that occur in circulating blood following a meal, such as glucose, amino acids and fatty acids can all regulate feeding behavior (the "static theories" of appetite regulation).

Messengers Controlling Appetite and Hoodia

Mediators or inhibitors (messengers) of feeding behavior include several endogenous hormones or peptides that can interact with different receptors in the brain or body. These regulators of feeding behaviors and energy balance include, but are not limited to, the following: melanocortin, leptin, bombesin, galanin, glucagon-like peptide 1, insulin and neuropeptide Y (NPY).

It has been proposed that steroidal glycosides present in Hoodia gordonii, and some related plant species, may act through a positive stimulant effect (agonist) on the melanocortin-4 receptor in the brain. It is recognized that a deficiency of melanocortin-4 receptors in animals causes gross obesity.

It is suggested that the agonist effect on this melanocartin-4 receptor triggers the satiety hormone cholecystokinin (CCK) and regulates the activity of NPY. While these proposals are quite plausible, they are unlikely to be a complete explanation of the effects of components of Hoodia on hunger, satiety, thirst, pleasure and feelings of "positive body energy".

Hoodia in the Brain and the Body

Animal studies with purified steroidal glycosides extracted from Hoodia, demonstrated that the direct injection of these active components of Hoodia reduced food intake in animals by a factor of up to 60% over a 24 hour period. There is no clear explanation about the precise mechanism of the effect of the components of Hoodia on increasing nerve cell activity in the hypothalamus. The researchers proposed that the effect of Hoodia on the brain was most likely a local effect. In other words, the observed effects on the brain were not thought to be due to the responses from the "whole body" and its various signals that control hunger, appetite and satiety.

There may be other mechanisms of action of Hoodia on appetite and the rat studies cannot be taken as a conclusive demonstration that the appetite suppressing effects of Hoodia are due only to a localized effect on the brain. Further research is required to illustrate the precise mechanism(s) of action(s) of Hoodia on hunger, appetite and feeling full.

Chapter Summary

The science of Hoodia gordonii is unraveling, but it remains underexplored. While extracts of Hoodia gordonii contain steroidal glycosides that exert effects on hunger and appetite, this may not be the only mechanism of action of Hoodia on appetite and energy balance? — vide infra.

CHAPTER 7

HOODIA IN HUMANS

Hoodia is Not a Magic Bullet: Needs for Lifestyle Change

It would be wrong to assume that Hoodia gordonii or its components could be a "magic bullet" for weight control. Hoodia affords the promise of assisting with behavior modification that could control calorie intake, which is the same as controlling energy intake into the body. Behavior modifications have emerged as very important factors in weight control. These programs are necessary for sustained weight control, and the promises of "this or that diet alone" for long term weight control has never been realized in the history of humankind. Behavior modification for weight control involves self-imposed restriction of eating habits, with reduced energy intake and many lifestyle changes. There must be resolve and commitment for weight control to be sustained.

Food Selections

There are very good reasons to watch the amount of fat intake in one's diet, with special reference to control over "bad fats". The notion of bad fats applies mainly to saturated fats found in association with animal protein or full-fat milk products. Modern concepts of healthy diets allow for the use of "good fats". Within the category of good fats are mainly the unsaturated or mono-unsaturated fats. In this context, the Mediterranean Diet has achieved increasing popularity because of its beneficial implications for health. It is reasonable to assume that most polyunsaturated fatty acids are healthy; and, in particular, Omega-3 fatty acids found in their active form in fish oils are quite desirable for inclusion in weight loss diets.

The Power of Omega-3 Fatty Acids

In brief, Omega-3 fatty acids found in fish oil or other marine products are among the most potent and versatile, health-giving natural substances known to humans. The Omega-3 fatty acids play a major role in cellular health and they are fundamental regulators of cardiovascular health, principle components of cell membranes, and they are key building blocks of the central nervous system. There are thousands of clinical studies that show the benefits of fish oil in common disorders such as cardiovascular disease, depression, attention deficit disorder, cancer prevention, and reduction of inflammatory disease.

While Omega3 fatty acid precursors are found in some vegetables, e.g., legumes (soy), and nuts, these precursors need to be converted to the active types of Omega-3 fatty acids that are readily found in fish oil concentrates. Many individuals have a reduced capacity to convert precursors of Omega-3 fatty acids into fatty acids that can be used effectively for health promotion by the body. Active fatty acids include EPA (eicosapentanoic acid) and DHA (docosahexanoic acid). The best sources of EPA and DHA are fish oils found mainly in cold water fish (mackerel, salmon, cod, etc.).

Many supplement users have relied on plant oils, such as flax seed oil, as a source of Omega-3 fatty acids in their diet, but it is important to know that plant oils, like flax seed oil, contain only Omega-3 precursor molecules. Therefore, I do not recommend vegetable sources of Omega-3 fatty acids as a reliable source of active omega-3 fatty acids that can be used for disease prevention o treatment purposes. There is a striking effect of Omega-3 fatty acids on reversing insulin resistance, and this makes fish oil an ideal companion for healthy weight loss and reduction of established cardiovascular and certain other disease risks that occur in obese individuals. Fish oil is a key nutraceutical in Syndrome X Nutritional Factors that can help combat Syndrome X (www.combat-syndromex.com). That said, there is a massive deficiency of Omega-3 fatty acids in Western diets, especially in the diet of youngsters.

Perhaps the readers of this book could reflect upon where the average American child gets Omega-3 fatty acids in their diet? The answer is that they do not often get them in their diet, and foods like fried fish fingers are not a good source of Omega-3 fatty acids. In fact, much of the fried food that we take in our diet, or permissively allow in our children's diet, contains damaged fats and disease-producing trans-fatty acids. While "Captain Crunch", "Mrs. Smith", and "Arthur Treacher" join other fast food friends in the purveyance of fish or reconstituted fish, they may be as much of a stranger to healthy fats, as some of the people eating their food.

Good This and Bad That in the Diet

I have purposely focused the introductory discussion in this chapter on dietary fats, so that I can dismiss the propaganda that all fat is healthy or unhealthy. I could have focused on "bad carbohydrates" (simple sugars) and "good carbohydrates" (complex sugars with fiber). Equally, I could have talked about "good proteins" and "bad proteins", if one wishes to subscribe to the notion that there are "bad proteins". I doubt that we can vilify types of protein, except to say that certain vegetable proteins have wide-reaching potential health benefits, e.g., soy protein (Holt, S *"The Soy Revolution"*, Dell Publishing, Random House, 2000). Again, I am referring to the possibility of altering macronutrient composition in the diet to have more healthy forms of macronutrients (fat, carbohydrate, and protein).

Having animal protein in one's diet a couple of days a week, with fish protein sources and vegetable protein sources on other days of the week, seems to make sense in achieving what people have poorly defined as "the balanced diet". I believe that soy protein has some major benefits in weight control because it is of low glycemic index, reduces blood cholesterol, may reduce blood pressure, and it possesses many other benefits for the overweight person (Holt, S *"The Soy Revolution"*, Dell Publishing, Random House, 2000). In fact, soy foods may be ideal foods for the pre-diabetic or diabetic individuals. I am not trying to turn Americans into vegetarians, but some movement away from "the meat and potatoes" dietary habits of Western society may improve overall health, while helping to control waistline expansion.

The Energy Equation of the Body

The body prepares itself for the unavailability of food (energy) by storing reserves in the form of glycogen and fats (triacylglycerols). Energy from food permits the body to do its daily chores of running the chemistry of life and letting humans move around in an intelligent manner.

Intelligence demands order. The body has many complicated ways of balancing its ability to "work", by exerting precise control mechanisms within the mind and body ("bodymind", or "mindbody"). No matter how clever a living system becomes at setting limits for energy balance, many things can go wrong with the delicate balance of "energy in and out" of the body. Excessive energy input into the body is stored as fat and we become obese. Lack of energy expenditure makes us fat. This is the relevance of the "energy equation of humankind".

Imperfect Laws of Physics, But Perfect Body Functions?

Nature has a way of outsmarting scientific principles that some may believe are "written in stone". Sometimes, I wonder if the makers of dietary supplements and weight control aids want to acknowledge scientific principles? The first law of thermodynamics states that energy cannot be created or destroyed. This means that energy or calories in the form of food do matter in the energy balance equations. In other words, "Calories Do Count".

A calorie is a calorie, is a calorie… and anyone who believes that "calories do not count" in weight control tactics should join the "Flat-Earth Society". While it is readily recalled that energy gets into the body in the form of food, it is often forgotten that most energy leaves the body in the form of heat due to processes of food breakdown (burning food or catabolism).

Although the first law of thermodynamics is easy to understand, the second law is a little more complex. The second law of thermodynamics tells us that all processes involving energy have a tendency to move in the direction of "maximum entropy". The notion of "entropy" provides a confusing circumstance for many people. Entropy is best understood as energy present in a system that cannot be made available to perform work that may be considered useful. Useful uses of energy include the energy support of the chemistry of life (basic body metabolism), movement (exercise), and energy that is required for breakdown and use of food eaten in the diet.

The simple way of looking at energy balance is to consider how changes in body energy stores relate to energy input and output from the body. Thus:

The difference between energy
intake (food eaten) and energy   =
out (utilization of food for energy)

Change in the energy stores
made by the body in the form
of glycogen and fat

Of course, food has its energy stored in special chemical configurations. The body has to take the energy out of food to put it in a form where it can use the energy. The nutrients in food contain the chemical configurations to which I refer. These configurations form carbohydrates, proteins and fats which are burned (oxidized) by the body to provide energy for use by the body. The healthy diet contains a balance of fat, carbohydrate and protein intake that assists in the achievement of energy balance (energy in and out of the body).

Our Partial Understanding of Energy Into and Out of the Body

The many factors that control energy balance in the body remain only partially understood. This means that the application of "concrete" physical principles can be expected to be rewarded only by unpredictable outcomes. In the "body-weight-set-point" theory, the body seems to defend a particular body weight even in the presence of energy deficits. To throw another "spanner in the works" is easy when one embraces the "body-weight-settling-point theory". The "settling theory" takes account of body weight and composition changes that occur over a human's lifetime. For example, women have more fat than men and a general increase in body weight occurs between the ages of thirty and sixty-five years, approximately. Thus, what the body may defend in early life as its own desired weight is subject to change over a lifetime. This explains why one diet cannot fit everyone's needs. The "one size fits all" concept in clothes is ridiculous and it is equally ridiculous if applied to diets.

In this discussion, we can add to the many variables that change body weight and body composition over our lifetime – almost ad infinitum. For example, appetite, total energy expenditure from the body and digestive function that assimilates food (energy) are all known to change with age. Aside from these "clever" scientific observations, economic factors change with age. Can our elderly population afford the best diet and what about our underprivileged sector of society?

Our society is not equipped to deal with the special nutritional needs of our elderly population and some of our elderly may not even know how to deal with their own needs. "Au contraire", how could we expect that our kids could handle their nutritional needs without education and appropriate oversight of their eating habits by parental guidance? Just watch "Kids' TV" and you may lose control over your own use of junk food! Junk food entices everyone to eat beyond their own satiety signals, as does alcohol (a relatively useless source of excess dietary energy!).

Does Hoodia Alter Energy Input or Output From the Body?

Suppression of appetite by Hoodia would be expected to cause a restriction of food intake. When feeding is restricted, changes can be expected to occur in both the energy input and output of the body. While changes in energy output as a consequence of reduced energy intake are small, over a period of time the body will tend to resist changes in body stores of energy. That said, Hoodia seems to be in itself somewhat "energizing". It remains to be seen if a person may become resistant to the appetite suppressing effects of Hoodia. Such resistance will promote the "plateau effect" in weight loss, where weight loss by the body is stubbornly opposed.

The output of energy from the body originates from carbohydrate, protein, and fat intake. The body draws upon these macronutrients for energy. Protein, fats and carbohydrate are supplied in the diet, or present in the body itself in storage forms, or as part of body structures. There is a certain priority that the body gives to oxidation (catabolism) of fats, carbohydrates and proteins. The major nutrients in our diet that cannot be stored are oxidized first by the body. Thus excess amino acids in the diet are oxidized before excess carbohydrates, which are, in turn, oxidized before excess fat.

Alcohol in the diet has a very high priority for oxidation, because it cannot be stored. It seems unlikely that Hoodia would exert any effect on altering the priority of oxidation of macronutrient substrates. Fat has a lower positioning in the body's election to burn fuel. It is reasonable to conclude that control of saturated fat intake in the diet would be advisable, when Hoodia is used as a weight control adjunct. It cannot be expected that Hoodia will alter a person's preference for certain foods in their diet, but this has not been researched in any detail.

Keeping Weight Off

The joy of losing weight in the short term is often accompanied by the disappointment of stubborn persistence of extra pounds (plateau), or weight regain in the intermediate to long term. This failure of weight loss strategies haunts the management of weight control. Some studies show that as many as 80% of dieters who are initially successful in losing body weight will regain their weight. Some dieters even finish up "fatter," after their "diet," in comparison to their status before their weight loss tactics. Plateau effects experienced during weight control or "yo-yo" weight regain is most likely to occur in individuals who have used "diet alone" to control their weight.

Although there are many behavioral aspects of weight control, that contribute to weight gain, there are also changes in body physiology during weight loss that will cause persistence of the flab, or its recurrence. We have learned that studies of people who have successfully controlled their weight show the importance of behavior modification, exercise and positive lifestyle changes in sustained weight loss. In recent times, the value of support groups in weight control strategies has become increasingly apparent, e.g., Weight Watchers. Psychological support for weight control is a key partner of behavior modification, for the successful "dieter".

Body Chemistry and Physiology That Resists Weight Control

Many changes in body physiology occur with weight loss. One important change with weight loss is a decrease in energy output by the body. It makes sense to recognize that a body carrying less weight would require less energy to operate. When weight loss occurs, about two thirds of the weight loss comes from fat loss, but about one third comes from muscles or fat-free body mass (FFM). The energy requirements to keep the chemistry of life going are known as the "resting metabolic rate". This important expenditure of energy in the resting metabolic rate is determined mainly by the FFM (fat-free mass) of the body. Diets that do not erode the fat-free mass (FFM) of the body are to be preferred in weight control strategies.

Understanding the changes in body physiology that occur with weight loss permits us to really understand the importance of exercise in sustained weight control. Of course, net energy intake should be controlled (lower calorie intake or "diet"), but increased physical activity plays a key role in sustained weight loss. If exercise ("getting on the move") is not addressed, then weight control may plateau or fail.

The degree to which energy output may decrease with weight loss varies greatly from one person to the other. This means that those people who have greater conservation of energy with weight loss will need more lifestyle changes for successful weight control. These changes involve more exercise. Individuals who conserve energy and conserve their fat stores are at an increased risk of the diet "yo-yo" or "plateau" effects.

It is reported that loss of weight in obese or overweight people causes a reduction of the ability of the body to "burn fat" (oxidize fat). If less fat is oxidized, while fat is still taken in the diet, there will be a greater tendency for fat to be stored in the body. This is one reason why low carbohydrate diets fail in many people.

Biological Activity of Hoodia in Humans

Phytopharm PLC and their scientific experts feel very strongly that it is the steroidal glycoside molecules in Hoodia that account for its overall beneficial effects in appetite control and weight loss. This conclusion may be premature, because there still is limited information on the mechanisms of the biological activity of Hoodia gordonii in humans. The rat's brain is quite different from the human brain and energy controlling mechanisms in the rat differ from those in humans.

Anyone observing rats while they feed must acknowledge that their feeding habits are very different than most humans. Furthermore, there is always a problem in projecting animal experiments into humans. While I believe that rats are thoughtful, feeling and intelligent beings, they do not come along with the "psychological baggage" or socio-behavioral complexities of humans. Rats do not eat in structured, social gatherings like humans, where social stimuli control eating behavior. Earlier, we discussed the complexities of the regulation of hunger, appetite and satiety in humans. One must take account of the great variation in how these sensations are experienced from one person to another.

Scientists have performed several complex clinical studies on Hoodia gordonii concentrates and extracts in humans. Not all of the scientific information has been reported, because much of the research is being used to contribute to the commercialization of the active fractions of Hoodia. The plan of commercialization involves the making of drugs or food additives. Currently, the most significant, reported human study of extracts of Hoodia was performed by researchers working with Phytopharm PLC (U.K.).

In these human experiments, a specific extract of Hoodia (P57) was used. Studies were performed in 20 obese individuals who were placed in a special environment, called a "metabolic unit". In this kind of "unit," close controls and observations can be undertaken on food intake and other body functions. The volunteers in those experiments were given either a "dummy pill" (placebo) or an active extract of Hoodia (P57). The volunteers were allowed to eat freely, read books, and watch TV. The subjects were able to generally lounge around, without any vigorous physical activity.

The individuals who received the P57 Hoodia extract reduced their calorie intake in their diets by about 1000 calories per day, of their own free will (Figure 4)! Food was plentiful for these people and readily available, but they reduced their food intake (energy into their bodies), when Hoodia was taken. Many individuals lost about 2 kilograms in weight over a couple of weeks and, as a group, the people receiving Hoodia had beneficial lowering of their blood sugar and blood triglycerides.

These results are striking and deserve much further investigation in longer term studies, with more detailed assessments of many body functions. These studies imply that components of Hoodia are active when given by mouth to humans. It is presumed that components of Hoodia reach the brain and act on energy balancing functions in the hypothalamus. Figure 4 summarizes this study in a schematic manner.

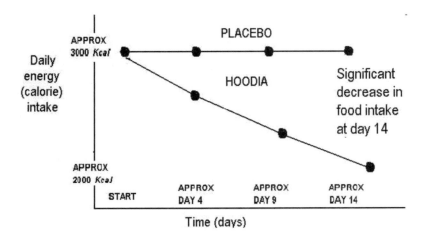

Figure 4: Schematic representation of the effect of Hoodia gordonii extracts on overweight humans. The lines represent trends in nine people on dummy pills (placebo) and nine people on Hoodia (Adapted from studies presented by Phytopharm, PLC, UK). Note: The data is presented with approximation, not complete accuracy, for illustrative purposes only of a biological effect that is the intellectual property of Phytopharm, PLC. Data such as these have not been generated with the use of any dietary supplement.

Uncontrolled Observations

There have been thousands of self reports of successful appetite and weight control with the oral administration of whole parts of Hoodia plants as a dietary supplement. Dietary supplements are made with dried Hoodia plant material, produced by variable methods of concentration. I believe that these findings of appetite control and weight loss with Hoodia supplements have not occurred by chance alone. Favorable results with Hoodia dietary supplements appear to be quite consistent among many individuals. It is not clear just how much steroidal glycoside content whole dried Hoodia plants or crude concentrates contain.

At the time of writing, there is only one form of Hoodia concentrate that has been used in a dietary supplement with significant customer satisfaction or reorder. This product is grown in South Africa and supplied to Syndrome X, Inc. and Natures Benefit Inc. of New Jersey. It is sold under the trademark Hoodia Supreme™ (www.hoodiasupreme.com) .

While there are many brands of Hoodia available over the internet for purchase, at the time of writing, no outcome observations have been reported. The author has been involved in collaborative research in testing a variety of material that has been sold as Hoodia gordonii and I regret to report that "fake material" has already entered the dietary supplement industry. This material has been imported from Mexico and China (caveat emptor).

Does Hoodia Work Only By Mechanisms Affecting The Brain?

Many individuals who have researched the appetite-suppressant activity of Hoodia and its components seem to be convinced that the only mechanism of action of Hoodia is on the central nervous system, specifically the hypothalamus. I believe that there may be other mechanisms of action of Hoodia on the body. My notions are supported by the complexities of controls of feeding behavior. I believe that Hoodia could affect appetite and weight control, by mechanisms other than the noted effects of Hoodia extracts on the brains of experimental animals.

It is unwise to assume that Hoodia and its components act only by one principle mechanism, because the control of hunger, appetite and satiety, is extraordinarily complex (intentional echolalia). Thus, there can be no firm conclusion at this stage, that steroidal glycoside molecules in Hoodia act alone in causing appetite suppression or other effects on body structures of function.

Some of the following discussions in this book are necessarily complex, and they may not be readily understood by individuals without biomedical knowledge or training. The simple message from this section of the book is that other mechanisms of action of Hoodia on the body may exist, and probably do exist. My opinion is supported by clinical observations of people who have taken Hoodia gordonii in whole forms or in concentrates.

I shall make it clear, later in this book, that products labeled as "extracts" and sold as dietary supplements are not true extracts of any specific fraction of Hoodia gordonii. What has been erroneously referred to as "extracts" of Hoodia on some dietary supplement labels should be redefined as "concentrates". Dietary supplements contain Hoodia gordonii, with varying contents of steroidal glycosides, protein, carbohydrate, fat, vitamins, and phytochemicals (phyto=plant). I believe that several, phytochemical components of Hoodia, with potential biological effects, may remain unidentified.

Alternative Explanations on the Mechanism of Action of Hoodia Gordonii

Steroidal glycosides have been identified in several different plant species. The action of these compounds on body structures and function remains quite underexplored in the medical sciences. For example, the thistle plant (Atractylis gummifera) contains steroidal glycosides that have been defined in some medical literature as toxic components of plants. Thistle-derived glycosides may cause depletion of glycogen in the body (Wogan GN, Marletta MA, 1985). Glycogen is a storage sugar that is used rapidly during any exercise. In fact, glycogen is often the first line of stored energy in the body. Glycogen is used rapidly as fuel during strenuous exercise. The steroidal glycoside components of thistle have been called "atractylosides".

While steroidal glycosides in the thistle plant have a chemical structure different from those found in Hoodia gordonii, there could be a common effect of steroidal glycosides on glycogen depletion? For the chemically-minded, the component of Hoodia that is believed to be a primary active component is an example of compounds called trirhabinosides. The chemical name reflecting the structure of this steroidal glycoside is 14-OH, 12-tigloyl pregnane steroidal glycoside (molecular weight, 1008). The molecular weight of this complicated molecule produces a size of molecule that could be well-absorbed by the gastrointestinal tract.

Steroidal glycosides have often a common chemical-core configuration, especially in relationship to the 14 hydroxyl (14-OH) substitution of the molecule. This shared chemical configuration makes the steroidal glycosides, found in Hoodia, chemically similar to other glycosides found in nature, otherwise referred to as "cardenolides". I shall try and keep the putative explanation of alternative mechanisms of action of Hoodia gordonii in a form that is readily understandable by many readers, but I cannot spare the readers the names of the chemicals involved. Simplication of technical issues sometimes corrupts information.

Glycogen, Energy and the Liver

Body stores of glycogen occur principally in the liver and muscle tissues of the body. The authors of the studies in rats, that described the effect of Hoodia gordonii on the brain (MacLean D, Lu-Guang L, 2004), did mention recent work suggesting that feeding habits in rats are directly related to the hepatic replenishment of energy in the form of ATP. The replenishment of ATP in the liver occurs as a consequence of feeding (Ji, H. Friedman, M.I. 1999). There is evidence in the medical literature that the liver can play a major role in the control of food intake. It appears that the liver collects information from changes in blood glucose concentration and fatty acid metabolism. This information is probably relayed from the liver to the brain by nerve connections (vagus nerves) or perhaps by unidentified hormonal signals.

The liver is the first organ in the body that nutrients encounter, after they are absorbed from digested food components. It appears probable that signals controlling food intake could even be triggered by the entry of nutrients into the veins that drains from the digestive tract into the liver (portal vein). In addition changes in nutrient contents in the blood or the brain following meals could cause signals that control food intake (Anderson G H, 1994). Following meals there are major changes in the concentration of many substances in the blood. These changes include variable blood concentrations of glucose, insulin, fatty acids, amino acids and hormones.

There are theories that link blood glucose concentration, blood insulin concentration and amino acid concentration as controllers of appetite and hunger. References to these complex events are present in the reference section of this book (Anderson G H, 1994, Novin D, 1985). The linkage between changes in the metabolism of body fuel (digested food) and appetite control have been reviewed in detail in the medical literature (Friedman MI, Rawson NE 1994).

Glucostatic Theories of Appetite Control

The change that occurs in blood glucose following meals has been identified as an important mechanism in the regulation of food intake. It is recognized that blood glucose is the number one source of cellular energy in the nervous tissue of the brain. The role of changes in blood glucose in the control of food intake has been referred to as "the glucostatic theory" of appetite control (Mayer J, 1955, Mayer J, 1980). The theories that relate to blood glucose and control of food intake involve the knowledge that glucose determines the availability of energy for the central nervous system and other body tissues. There is no doubt that glucose levels in the blood are closely monitored by body structures, including the hypothalamus of the brain.

Over the past 20 years the glucostatic theory of food, intake control has been evaluated in both animals and humans. In experiments using rats, it is known that quite small and even transient reductions in blood glucose, lasting only a matter of few minutes, are associated with changes in feeding habits (Campfield LA, Smith FJ, 1990). In fact these experiments in rats show that reductions in blood glucose concentrations by a factor of approximately 12 %, lasting for approximately 18 minutes, cause feeding activity in experimental animals. If one were to assume that a break down of glycogen in liver or muscle tissue causes transient increases in blood glucose, then one would assume that transient increases in blood glucose may stop feeding behavior.

The suggestions that steroidal glycosides may cause the breakdown of glycogen in the liver or muscle implies, by inference, that this putative action of steroidal glycosides may be responsible, at least in part, for an inhibition of feeding behavior. While this effect on glycogen breakdown in the body is an apparent with steroidal glycosides from the thistle plant, such proposals have not been made concerning a similar effect that may occur with steroidal glycosides found in Hoodia gordonii, or other related species of plant.

The evidence for changes in blood glucose and feeding in humans is apparent in experiments where individuals are studied in an environment where they are isolated from time cues that may stimulate eating (Campfield LA, Smith FJ, Rosenbaum M, et al, 1992). I believe that Hoodia may cause direct fluctuations blood glucose, by direct or indirect mechanisms, and this requires scientific investigation. In humans, it is apparent that small declines in blood glucose increase the intensity of hunger and "requests" for meals in individuals who are studied in an environment where they are isolated from time cues for meals (Campfield LA, et al., 1992).

Effects of Hoodia Unrelated to Appetite?

Much can be made of the importance of blood glucose and feeding habits in animals and humans. My assertions on the importance of these issues gains support from observations on the effects of Hoodia gordonii, that are unrelated to effects on appetite or hunger or satiety. It is known that the San Bushmen described Hoodia gordonii as a plant that not only suppresses appetite, but it has an energizing effect that is quite reproducible.

I have experienced the energizing effect of Hoodia gordonii myself after taking a dietary supplement containing whole Hoodia plant called, Hoodia Supreme™ (www.hoodiasupreme.com). In addition, several individuals who have used this dietary supplement report an energizing effect, in addition to an effect of appetite suppression. Thus, the folklore history of the energizing effect of Hoodia gordonii has been replaced in open label observations of the use of Hoodia gordonii in a dietary supplement (Hoodia Supreme™). I do not state these findings as complete evidence of alternative mechanisms of action of Hoodia gordonii, because these observations require further study. However, my observations are consistent with folklore history and the ethnobotanical use of Hoodia gordonii and related succulent plants. However, dietary supplements made with Hoodia gordonii may not work in all people.

In summary, I propose that the energizing effects of Hoodia gordonii may be due to a temporary, perhaps even short lived, rise in blood glucose that results from glycogen breakdown in peripherals tissues, caused by Hoodia gordonii. It is fascinating how these folklore observations of the use of Hoodia as a food by the San-bushmen seem to fit with scientific studies or "observations". Therefore, I propose that Hoodia gordonii may have effects, other than those occurring as direct consequences of the actions of the components of Hoodia gordonii on the central nervous system.

Hoodia: An Aphrodisiac?

Other folklore observations on the effects of Hoodia gordonii have been somewhat ignored by scientists. The San Bushmen in South Africa reported that Hoodia gordonii may have an aphrodisiac effect and even other pleasurable effects. In recent, elegant scientific studies, it has been demonstrated that the human brain produces and or metabolizes plant compounds. This is fascinating work which supports many of my beliefs in natural medicine. It seems clear to me that the evolution of humankind, in association with the plant kingdom, must have influenced our complicated body chemistry, over a period of many thousands of years.

In December 2004, the revered journal, Scientific American, published an article by Roger A. Nicoll and Bradley E Alger entitled "The Brain's Own Marijuana". In brief, the nervous system engages in the natural production and use of chemical compounds that are closely related to chemicals found in the Cannabis plant (marijuana). Marijuana use spells pleasure, pain control, alterations in memory, and alterations in appetite for many people who use this illicit drug. Later in this chapter, I speculate on the potential direct or indirect effects on signals in the brain that operate on the basis of "plant compounds" (chemicals of Nature). After all, marijuana is highly effective promoting appetite in people with digestive upset caused by toxic drugs (e.g. chemotherapy) or serious diseases, such as AIDS (Acquired Immune Deficiency Syndrome) - vide infra. Table 5 shows signals to the brain that alter eating behavior or control food intake.

CHEMICAL MESSAGES
Blood glucose, amino acid and fatty acid levels
Storage deposit signals mediated by insulin, glycogen, leptin and ketone bodies (Ketosis induced by carbohydrate restricted diets, e.g., Atkins' Diet)

MESSAGES FROM THE GUT
Gastrointestinal hormones: e.g., cholecystokinin, gastric inhibitory peptide, bombesin, etc.
Nerve relays, e.g., Vagus nerve

MESSAGES FROM THE ENVIRONMENT
Social circumstances, sight, taste, smell of food, stress, pleasure, etc.

TABLE 5: Examples of signals to the brain that alter eating behavior or control food intake.

Hoodia, Insulin and Metabolic Syndrome X

Changes in blood glucose are invariably associated with changes in blood insulin; and it is recognized that changes in blood insulin alter hunger, appetite, food intake and weight gain. Circulating blood insulin causes tissues to "build". In other words, it is an anabolic hormone that causes glucose uptake by many tissues; and it causes the uptake of amino acids by certain body tissues. There is no doubt that high circulating levels of blood insulin are strongly associated with increased appetite, hunger, food intake and the promotion of obesity (Schwartz MW, Figlewicz DP, Woods SC, et al 1993, Heller RF, Heller RF, 1994).

Increased circulating blood insulin (hyperinsulinemia) is the fundamental basis of the metabolic Syndrome X, which links insulin resistance to the variable occurrence of obesity high blood pressure and high blood cholesterol, with high blood triglycerides. Cravings for carbohydrates in some individuals, especially those who are obese, is probably related to "changes" in blood glucose concentration as well as "prevailing" blood glucose concentrations, which in turn are linked to changes in levels of insulin in the blood.

It is clear that insulin has some effects on feeding activity, by actions in the central nervous system. However, the actual origin of insulin in the brain is not well understood and insulin does not freely enter the nervous system from the general blood circulation in the body. Insulin acts within the nervous system to actually reduce food intake, but these observations are based largely on animal experiments (Gerozissis M, Orosco M, Rouch C, et al, 1993, McGowan MK, Andrews KM, Grossman SB, 1992).

Brain Centers and Messenger Molecules

There are centers in the brain that use novel messenger molecules that effect feeding behavior (Table 6). For example the arcuate nucleus of the brain manufactures or uses neuropeptide Y as a messenger to stimulate feeding in a potent manner. (Schwartz MW, et al., 1993). One may continue to see just how complicated central nervous system controls of appetite, hunger and satiety really are! For example if the brain levels of insulin change due to alterations in circulating insulin concentrations in the general circulation, because of reduced dietary intake of calories, one would expect an increased production of neuropeptide

Y within the arcuate nucleus of the brain. This would be expected to result in a powerful stimulus to promote food intake. This may indeed be the case (Schwartz MW, et al., 1993).

MESSENGER SUBSTANCES THAT INCREASE FOOD INTAKE
Chemicals that transmit messages among nervous tissue include: gamma aminobutyrate, catecholamines, growth hormone releasing factor

Hormones or peptides including: galanin, peptide YY, opioids, endo-cannabinoids, NYP, endorphins, enkephalins, etc.

MESSENGER SUBSTANCES THAT INHIBIT FOOD INTAKE
Neurotransmitters including: serotonin, dopamine, GABA, etc.
Hormones as peptides such as CCK, bombesin, somatostatin, corticotropic releasers, etc.

Table 6: Messenger molecules in the body or central nervous system that control, start, or stop food intake. Messenger controls of feeding are extraordinarily complex.

Aminostatic and Lipostatic Theories of Feeding Behavior

While I have concentrated on the role of glucose and insulin in altering hunger and appetite, there is evidence that fat intake or protein intake may also control these body sensations, relevant to feeding (Tables 5 and 6). Alternations in plasma amino acid concentration can effect feelings of appetite in humans (Mellinkoff SM, Frankland M, Boyle D, et al, 1956). This is called the "aminostatic theory". This theory implies that hunger and appetite are controlled by the ability of the brain, and perhaps other parts of the body, to sense changes in the blood concentrations of certain amino acids (Gietzen DW, 1986, Geitzen DW, 1993).

Challenging Current Knowledge of Hoodia's Actions

The principle reason why I challenge the current scientific findings behind Hoodia gordonii, in terms of its mechanism of action as an appetite suppressant, is the clear knowledge that any scientific report that focuses on a single system for the control of food intake must be questioned (see tables 5 and 6). Readers who understand the complexity of control of food intake must treat claims of single mechanism of actions of Hoodia gordonii with utmost skepticism, without further rigorous scientific studies.

Let it be clear that the effects of Hoodia gordonii, or any extracts of this plant, on prevailing blood levels of amino acids, glucose, or fatty acids, are underexplored. I have avoided too much discussion about the role of fat intake in controlling appetite, but it is well known that fat intake involves behavioral responses and hormonal responses that cause satiety. For example, fat intake in the diet releases the hormone cholecystokin (CCK). The hormone CCK is a well recognized satiety signal that provides a powerful message to interrupt eating. Furthermore, CCK can slow stomach emptying and contribute to the triggering of stretch receptors in the stomach that, in turn, give their own signals for satiety.

I caution readers again that the complex systems that regulate food intake in animals are not exactly the same as those that operate in humans (Tables 5 and 6). This difference in regulating systems for energy balance is well documented in genetic studies in morbidly obese humans (Hamilton BS, Paglia D, Kwan AYM, et al 1995). Scientists do not fully understand how genetic material in the body acts to regulate obesity in humankind. Genetic controls of hunger and appetite and associated body functions compound an understanding of the mechanism of the effects of appetite suppressants. Could it be that San bushmen and their relatives are genetically programmed to be more susceptible to the effects of Hoodia? This is doubtful, but interesting.

Plants Talk to the Brain

Humankind has evolved in a biosphere of massive and complex communication among living organisms. It seems logical to conclude that the plant kingdom must have exerted major effects on the human evolutionary process. The reported findings that compounds in the plant kingdom affect body structures and functions is the basis of traditional, natural and modern medicine. Indeed, it is known that almost every synthetic pharmaceutical used in disease treatment or prevention, can be found in one form or another in Nature. While the actions of herbs or other botanicals on the body is accepted as obvious, it is not easy to comprehend why plants would contain chemicals that are used directly or indirectly in the messenger systems of the brain (brain signals).

Examples of the use of plant-related compounds in the communication systems of the brain include: opium (morphine) and endocannabinoids (endogenous cannabinoids). Morphine (opium) is found in the poppy and cannabinoids are found in marijuana (Cannabis sativa). The chemical compounds called "cannabinoids" get their name from the plant known as "Cannabis", otherwise referred to as marijuana, hash, hashish, ganja, bhang, weed, etc.

The isolation of morphine from poppies led to research that explained the multiple actions of crude poppy extracts on the human body. These actions included a propensity for addiction, pain control, mind alteration, and "pleasure promotion". There are receptors for "morphine-like" compounds in many animals and living organisms. These are often called "opiate receptors" that can react with specific "molecules of emotion" (Dr. Candace Pert's Aphorism).

Following the discovery of opiate receptors in humans, came the discovery that humankind makes their own opium-like (morphine-like) compounds called "opiods". These opiods include brain messengers called enkephalins and endorphins. With this background, one can begin to understand how plant chemicals, like opium or morphine, can act on the central nervous system.

In simple terms, plant chemicals like morphine (opioids) latch on to the brain receptors that are present to react to the body's own opiods (enkephalins and endorphins). Opioid receptors are an important part of brain signals that affect feelings, sensations, appetite and behavior, etc. In recent times, the discovery of receptors in the brain that respond to cannabinoids has cast further light on the phenomenon of *"plants talking to the human brain"*.

Ancient medical disciplines such as Ayurvedic medicine and Traditional Chinese Medicine recognized the ability of the poppy (with its content of opium) to exert mind altering, pain-relieving and other effects on the body. In a similar manner, the ancient tribe of the San bushmen of South Africa recognized the hunger suppressing, energizing, pleasing and aphrodisiac effects of Hoodia gordonii. The difference among these phenomena is that opiods from the poppy and cannabinoids from Cannabis (marijuana) have receptors on nerve cells in the human brain to act upon, whereas no specific receptors have been identified in the brain for the putative, active constituents of Hoodia gordonii (the steroidal glycosides).

Hoodia Talks to the Brain

Although components of Hoodia gordonii are clearly "talking to the brain", when they reduce hunger and appetite, their "pathway" of communication may be less direct than the pathway of communication made by other plant-related substances, such as opioids or cannabinoids. I reiterate that there is no evidence that the human brain has receptor sites for steroidal glycosides or that the brain uses these kinds of molecules in its own signaling systems (messenger molecules). However, a commonality exists among the effects of morphine (opioids), cannabinoids, and components of Hoodia gordonii (presumed steroidal glycosides) on specific brain functions, most notably "pleasure" and "feeding" behavior. These similarities between the overall effects of "three kinds" of plants that can talk to the brain raises the need for some more speculation on the mechanisms of action of plant compounds on the central nervous system.

Brain Messengers and Final Common Pathways

The brain has to "integrate" information from multiple sources, make intelligent "decisions" and give instructions through final common pathways. In these acts, the brain uses chemical signals that cause chemical events. These events act in turn to cause nervous tissue to send their messages by impulse generation. I propose that the three groups of plant compounds that are being discussed (opioids, cannabinoids and steroid glycosides) may have considerable interdependence in their actions on the brain, and perhaps even interdependence in their chemical mode of actions, by direct or indirect mechanisms.

Attempts to work out how opioids or cannabinoids exert complicated effects on brain and body functions have taken more than a century. Despite this extensive research, our knowledge of the effect of Hoodia gordonii on the brain is quite embryonic.

Complicated research involving receptor chemistry in the brain has elucidated some mechanisms of action of plant compounds that talk to the brain. These discussions are beyond the scope of this book, but it is my belief that components of Hoodia gordonii may share, at least indirectly, communication pathways with opioids or cannabis. The logic behind my proposal is the shared action of poppies, cannabis, and Hoodia on feeding activity. It is with humility that I hope that this is not too bold a leap of logic?

In brief, morphine exerts a major influence on appetite and it induces satiety. Morphine (opium) causes almost complete, temporary delays in stomach emptying and it has central effects that can reduce or promote nausea and vomiting. Opium addicts do not eat well and they have a poor appetite, both of which lead to wasting of the body and the wasting-syndrome of drug addiction. Cannabis can have a similar effect to opiods, and cannabinoids enjoy effective use as drugs that suppress nausea and stimulate appetite in many people. This action of cannabinoids has led to the attempt to develop drugs that can block cannabinoid receptors and suppress appetite.

There have been some early clinical trials on cannabinoid-receptor-blocking-drugs that appear to reduce appetite, but many side effects have been encountered from these early drug development projects that involve involve "cannabinoid blockers". Research on the development of and anti-obesity drug from "cannabinoid-blockers" used a chemical agent that blocked the CB1 receptor in the brain. This receptor responds to endocannabinoids (Nicoll RA, et al, 2004).

The scientific issues that surround brain receptor chemistry and functions are more complex than can be discussed in this book. There are many intermediary signals involved in how plants talk to the brain. Expanding the knowledge of "this dialogue of nature" provides a legion of exciting possibilities for the development of compounds or the isolation of natural substances that can control appetite, digestive upset, pain and even pleasure.

CHAPTER 8

HOODIA ENTERS COMMERCE

Confusion Prevails

Several patents have been filed on Hoodia gordonii and its components in a manner that is centered around the effect of Hoodia gordonii on appetite suppression. Patents are usually filed as a prelude to commercialization, with a clear intent to protect an invention. There has been much debate about the ability of businesses to file "solid patents" on natural products. The perceived inability of commercial organizations to patent and protect natural products as medicines is one of the main reasons why there is relatively little financial investment in research of natural medicines, compared with synthetic drugs.

I have discussed matters of developing drugs or treatments from nutrients, herbs and botanicals in detail in the medical literature (Holt, S, Natural Product Development and Use, in Pharmacy Ventures, Pharmaceutical Discovery and Development and Drug Delivery, Companies Reports, Oxford, UK, 2001). Suffice it to say that components of botanicals or other remedies of natural origin can be subject readily to a patent filing, especially if they are presented in an extracted chemical form or in synthetic versions of extracted chemicals. However, a patent on a whole botanical for a specific use is always questionable, especially if "prior art" exists. "Prior art" means simply "prior widespread knowledge of the proposed invention".

Prior art is often present with remedies of natural origin in folklore, traditional medical disciplines and recorded ethnobotanical use of plants. This appears to be the prevailing circumstance with Hoodia gordonii and related species, but one may expect some members of the legal profession to argue to the contrary. In fact, the San bushmen argued strongly for the case of "prior art," when they questioned the filing of patents by the South African CSIR on the use of extracts of Hoodia as an appetite suppressant. This research agency in Pretoria,

South Africa, filed patents on the use of steroidal glycosides in Hoodia gordonii, specifically as an appetite suppressant.

It appears that the San bushmen had a case against the CSIR patents because they were awarded royalties from Hoodia patent holders after legal altercations, upon information and belief. A discussion of some aspects of the patents that have been filed on the components of Hoodia is worthwhile, but "who owns what" may be challenged in the future, especially if commercial interests cross pathways in revenue generation – enter the lawyers?

Observations On "Hoodia Patents"

Perhaps the most significant patent filed on Hoodia is US Patent No. US6,376,657B1 by Van Heerden F.P. and others. This patent has an assignment of rights to the Pretoria-based CSIR, a quasi-government research agency of South Africa. This patent describes in detail a pharmaceutical composition or compositions which contain appetite suppressing extracts that can be obtained from plants of the families Trichocaulon or Hoodia (gordonii and lugardii). This patent makes specific reference to a formula of a steroidal glycoside molecules. In addition, it describes techniques for extraction of certain compounds from the plants in question. Also, it describes a process for synthesizing the alleged active components of Hoodia and related analogues or other "steroidal glycoside-like compounds".

The inventions in this patent extend themselves to foodstuff or drinks that could contain effective quantities of steroidal glycosides. Dietary supplements are not specifically mentioned in the patent.

The proposed effects of the Hoodia in this patent relate the potential development of "foodstuffs" that may have an ability to suppress appetite. The patent indicates that the active ingredients may be of a chemical structure of a steroidal glycoside that can be found in plants of the genus (family) Trichocaulon or Hoodia. The patent focuses somewhat on the species Hoodia gordonii, but it also refers to other species including: Trichocaulon officinale, Trichocaulon piliferum or species of the genus Hoodia (Hoodia gordonii, Hoodia currorii, and Hoodia lugardii). Researchers have looked further into the properties of Hoodia extracts that may be beneficial for health. These promises of even more health benefits from Hoodia gordonii are not generally known to the public – vide infra.

Hoodia Has Other Potential Benefits?

In a US Patent dated Dec. 3, 2002, researchers from the US and South Africa describe an invention where Hoodia components may have multiple benefits for digestive health, by causing reductions in acid secretion by the stomach (Hakkin J, et al, US Patent No.: 6,488,967). This patent describes a method of treating disease or disorders of the gastrointestinal tract, using extracts of plants of the genus Hoodia or Trichocaulon or related chemical compounds.

It appears that one or more of the appetite suppressing compounds present in Hoodia may be quite effective in reducing the secretion of acid by the stomach. This effect of Hoodia components on acid secretions by the stomach seems to be present at higher doses of the Hoodia extract. For example, injections of specific types and doses of Hoodia extracts into rats has been recorded to inhibit gastric acid secretion by a factor of up to 43%.

These effects of Hoodia components on acid output from the stomach raises possibility that they may have a use in the treatment of acid-related digestive disorders, such as: reflux esophagitis, gastro-esophageal reflux, peptic ulcer, non-ulcer dyspepsia and even damage to the linings of the upper digestive tract caused by ulcerogenic drugs (e.g., non-steroidal anti-inflammatory drugs, NSAID). This digestive benefit of Hoodia is a wonderful coincidence in clinical practice. Overweight people have a higher incidence of acid-related digestive upset, especially gastroesophageal reflux disease (GERD). What about the idea of controlling appetite and losing weight, while taking care of indigestion?

How is Hoodia To Be Used?

The traditional use of Hoodia gordonii for its appetite suppressant effect involved the eating of whole, fresh plants or perhaps dried plants. Flowers, roots, and spiky skin on the plant were not eaten readily by anyone, including the hardy San bushmen. The natural use of Hoodia involved cutting open the skin, and eating or drinking the flesh and sap of the plant. In fact, several TV correspondents have taken the plant in this traditional form. These newscasters, along with others, comment upon its bitterness, and almost immediate effects on appetite suppression. It is clear that Hoodia gordonii cannot be taken in this fresh form by many consumers. Therefore, the Hoodia plant in South Africa has been processed by drying the plant and producing powder or concentrates that can be used in dietary supplements, or perhaps added to food.

The use of Hoodia in a dietary supplement is closer to the traditional use of Hoodia than the isolation of certain extracts of Hoodia (steroidal glycosides). Although recent scientific experiments seem to support that specific fractions or extracts of Hoodia gordonii are responsible for its major effects on appetite, it is not safe to assume that other ingredients within Hoodia do not contribute to its many effects in humans. The precedent for the safety of taking Hoodia rests with the use of the whole plant, not with the use of extracts such as steroidal glycosides.

In this book, I have proposed that there may be several alternative mechanisms of action of Hoodia in the control of feeding behavior; and one may need to invoke other explanations of its mechanisms of action in order to explain the reports of its energizing capabilities and its effects in the promotion of pleasure and sexual activity. Even the extracts of Hoodia gordonii, that have been proposed in patents to be the active constituents of the plant, are known to have effects on areas of the body other than the brain, e.g., the effect of components of Hoodia on acid secretion by the stomach. Several proponents of natural medicine have developed a consensus that the way to go with Hoodia is to take the whole plant, without its flowers or roots. This way of preparing Hoodia gordonii as a bulk reagent for use in dietary supplements seems prudent, given the current level of scientific knowledge.

The rational use of Hoodia in a dietary supplement would involve the taking of a powder, capsule, or tablet of material produced from the whole plant. There seems to be no doubt that biologically active constituents in Hoodia are regularly absorbed from the digestive tract. In other words, the oral ingestion of Hoodia plant would be expected to have effects on the body similar to those described by the San bushmen, as long as the components of Hoodia that are responsible for its effects are not destroyed during processing.

There are many possible ways of processing the Hoodia plant. Some of these methods of processing have been disclosed in patents, and some involve the arbitrary use of drying techniques, sterilization techniques, and in some cases, the use of chemicals to concentrate components of Hoodia.

Criticisms of Hoodia as a Dietary Supplement

Scientists and members of corporate organizations that are involved in drug development strategies with steroidal glycosides are highly critical of the use of Hoodia gordonii in a "natural manner". These individuals consider the production of bulk, whole plant material will result in an inactive dietary supplement, because of a failure to concentrate steroidal glycosides during processing. Furthermore, it is clear, that any attempts to make steroidal glycoside concentrates or fractions could be readily interpreted as an infringement of patents held by major business corporations. It is apparent that these corporations are fixated upon the development of food additives or drugs that rely upon concentration of the steroidal glycosides in Hoodia gordonii.

Spokespersons for the companies involved in the licensing and transfer of patent rights for Hoodia gordonii have been openly critical of the development of dietary supplements. These "drug advocates" argue that many such supplements are without any useful activity. It is important to realize that the companies that file the patents, and government researchers in South Africa, did achieve positive outcomes with the use of crude concentrates of Hoodia gordonii, and they identified what they believed to be the active fraction. These researchers saw consistent biological activity of Hoodia as they "honed in" on the steroidal glycoside molecules, found in Hoodia. On the one hand, patent holders criticize the use of the whole plant or crude concentrates, but on the other hand, there is evidence that these more natural forms of Hoodia can be effective in biological systems, by altering feeding behavior in animals and humans.

There is always a big problem with drug development pathways, when it comes to disclosure of experimental results. To take care of proprietary interests, and perhaps other interests, a lot of research done during "drug development" is not reported freely in the medical literature. I cannot state with any confidence that there are observations on the mechanism of action of Hoodia that have not been disclosed by several researchers. In fact, one would expect selective disclosure of information of Hoodia research by companies that are trying to commercialize their intellectual property during drug discovery.

Looking at Material Used in Dietary Supplements

My colleagues and I have analyzed batches of material that is alleged to come from South Africa. The material supplied by some companies in the dietary supplement industry varies dramatically in its appearance and composition. Some tested material, labeled as Hoodia, was imported from China. This "Chinese Hoodia" is not likely to be Hoodia gordonii, and it was found to contain unacceptable levels of heavy metals and bacteria. The easiest way to spot quality Hoodia gordonii material is to examine the overall composition of the bulk material. Table 7, below, gives product identification measurements expressed both in weight in grams per hundred grams, and weight in five grams for principle constituents.

Attempts are being made to measure steroidal glycoside content in bulk material that is available for use in dietary supplements in the USA. The data disclosed in this section of the book was supplied by Stella Labs, Inc. of Washington Township, NJ and this material is a 20:1 concentrate from drying procedures, it is not an extract. Other information related to this product is displayed below in Table 7, courtesy of Stella Labs, Inc.

Hoodia gordonii 20:1	Specifications
Botanical Name:	Hoodia gordonii
Family	Asclepiadaceae
Appearance	Light green to brownish powder
Part used	Aerial stem
Origin	South Africa
pH	5.41
Ash	3.95%
Extract ratio	20:1

Microbiological Analysis:	
Total Plate Count:	<10,000 cfu/g
Yeast:	100 cfu/g
Mold:	100 cfu/g
E. Coli	Negative
Pseudomonas:	Negative
Salmonella:	Negative
Coag. Pos Staphylococcus	Negative

Heavy Metals <10ppm **As** <2ppm **Pb** <3ppm

The bulk material that has been studied by Stella Labs in is supplied by Synhealth Corporation of South Africa, which has entered into a world-wide, exclusive supply agreement with Stella Labs of NJ.

Variability in Cost of Hoodia: Implications

It must be expected that not all dietary supplements, containing or labeled as Hoodia, will be created in an egalitarian manner. At the time of writing, I could find evidence of approximately 24 different brands of Hoodia supplements on the internet. The dosage of Hoodia in these supplements is quite variable, but the dosage listed can sometimes be quite irrelevant, because in some cases the material used to make the supplement is not Hoodia gordonii, and bulk material may have been "cut" or adulterated by various means. Based on open-label observations, it would appear that an average effective dose of high quality, Hoodia gordonii material is 400mg taken once or twice daily before main meals in one day. My suggestion of this average dosage only applies to high quality, Hoodia that is imported from South Africa. High quality material is obtained from reliable growers and processors with permits provided by the South African government (www.hoodiasupreme.com).

Not only is there major inconsistency in recommended doses of Hoodia supplements, there is considerable difference in price. Prices range from less than $20 to more than $80 per bottle and the commonest bottle counts of capsules or tablets in Hoodia supplements are 30 or 60.

One must be quite skeptical about inexpensive dietary supplements containing Hoodia because pure, quality bulk Hoodia gordonii costs on average at least $300 per kilo to purchase for the manufacturing of dietary supplements. Variations of price in bulk material that is called "Hoodia" have been reported in recent times in a range from US $35 per kilogram to more than US $700 per kilogram. When prices of anything do not make sense, one must assume that there is great difference in the commodity in question.

The cost of high quality Hoodia and its probable, future problems with sustainable supplies have prompted some dietary supplement manufacturers to use smaller dosages or combinations of other weight loss supplements with Hoodia gordonii.

Hoodia Alone or In Combination

Modern dietary supplement technology often involves a combination of nutrients, herbs or botanicals that may act together in an additive manner (synergy). The synergistic use of dietary supplements that may promote weight control or combat the metabolic syndrome X makes much sense. There have been suggestions that Hoodia gordonii may be very valuable in the management of the metabolic syndrome X, at least in relationship to its potential ability to help with weight loss. These circumstances have encouraged me to incorporate Hoodia gordonii into a group of dietary supplements that I have termed "Syndrome X Nutrional Factors®." The question remains: *What would be ideal synergistic ingredients for use in weight control supplements with Hoodia gordonii?*

The selection of synergistic ingredients in a supplement containing Hoodia gordonii should not detract from the obvious advantages of Hoodia. Hoodia gordonii does not contain any stimulants and individuals who have proposed the use of strong stimulants to suppress appetite, in combination with Hoodia are misguided. Some patents have been filed on the combination of strong stimulant supplements to be used in combination with Hoodia, but this situation defeats the clear benefits of the non-stimulant, appetite suppressing-effects of Hoodia.

While patents have been filed on combinations of other natural substances to be used with Hoodia in dietary supplements, at the time of writing the patent fillings were pending and not granted. As a "rule of thumb", any drug or natural substances that is strong enough to suppress appetite, by a stimulant effect, is strong enough to raise blood pressure and present cardiovascular risks. Heart attack and stroke can occur with some stimulants and this is why ephedra (ma huang) was removed from the dietary supplement market, as a weight control aid. I have no reason to believe that synephrine, contained in Citrus aurantium, is much safer than ephedra. In brief, I could not propose combinations of potent "stimulating" natural compounds with Hoodia.

It would make sense to use natural substances that may overcome insulin resistance with Hoodia gordonii. Such natural substances include alpha lipoic acid, chromium, vanadium and selected antioxidants. Of particular benefit may be the use of Hoodia with viscous dietary fiber, such as oat beta glucan (hydrocolloid fractions of oat bran). Indeed, I have reviewed a number of natural agents that may help combat syndrome X in three books that I have written (Holt S, Combat Syndrome X, Holt S, et al, Nutrional Factors for Syndrome X, Holt S, Enhancing Low Carb Diets, www.wellnesspublishing.com).

I believe that a particularly valuable combination of dietary supplements for weight control are high quality Hoodia gordonii whole plant combined with coffee bean extracts. Coffee consumption has had a "rocky history", in terms of its health implications. However, coffee is major source of substances that may benefit individuals involved in weight control tactics. Coffee contains caffeine that has the unwanted action of reducing sensitivity to insulin. This effect of caffeine is contrary to guidelines of promoting insulin sensitivity to combat the metabolic syndrome X. However, coffee presents some health giving substances and it can be used in a decaffeinated form.

Coffee contains well absorbed polyphenol compounds and the phenol "chlorogenic acid" has very favorable effects on carbohydrate metabolism. Not only is chlorogenic acid a powerful antioxidant, it acts to reduce the absorption of glucose into the body. Furthermore, it inhibits body enzymes in a way that reduces sugar output from the liver. Thus, coffee has emerged with a promise of benefit in overcoming"sugar problems" or glucose intolerance. A recent study by Van Dam R M and Feskens E J M, reported in 2002, indicated that coffee consumption was associated with a reduced risk of developing Type II diabetes mellitus.

The science supporting the value of chlorogenic acid in healthy weight control and potential combat against the metabolic syndrome X is strong. Chlorogenic acid can inhibit an enzyme that is part of a system of enzymes called glucose-6-phosphatase.This extract of coffee bean has been identified as a specific inhibitor of glucose-6-phosphate translocase. This specific enzyme will tend to reduce the high rates of output of glucose from the liver that are often present in individuals with obesity, the metabolic syndrome X and Type II diabetes mellitus. I have observed excellent outcome in weight control, and reversal of blood lipid problems with the combination of coffee bean extract containing chlorogenic acid and Hoodia gordonii. I have proposed this unique combination of natural compounds as a new invention (patent).

One powerful aspect of the combination of chlorogenic acid or other phenolic components of coffee with Hoodia gordonii, relates to a complimentary beneficial action on fat storage and lipolysis. Well conducted animal studies imply that chlorogenic acid is able to cause insulin sensitivity, resulting in improved glucose tolerance and decreased blood lipids (cholesterol) (Rodriguez de Sotillo D.V., Hadley M, 2002). In these studies, genetically obese rats showed improvements in glucose tolerance combined with reductions in insulin concentrations that appear to decrease the synthesis of lipids by the liver. These factors would be expected to favorably alter some metabolic problems found in the obese individual with syndrome X.

One very useful addition to a healthy weight control diet is green tea polyphenols. Not only is green tea considered to be a cancer preventive and anti inflammatory agent, it has beneficial effects on glucose metabolism that could compliment the actions of chlorogenic acid or Hoodia (www.greenteamax.com).

Dietary Supplements Touted for Weight Loss

The dietary supplement industry has experienced a number of commercial failures with weight loss aids. Furthermore, many fad diets have fizzled in their importance and not delivered their promises. The most popular of all weight loss aids was ephedra [ma huang]. Ephedra was removed from the dietary supplement market because it was believed to contribute to heart attacks and strokes, among other problems. In the wake of the "ephedra controversy," the dietary supplement industry is reaching constantly for new natural substances that may assist in weight control.

While some of the many supplements, touted as weight control agents, possess some advantages, there is no compelling evidence that many of these newly "touted" supplements can provide stand-alone management of weight control. In fact, the evidence for their benefits remains dubious in many cases. The exciting thing about Hoodia gordonii is a combination of the longstanding precedent of safety and effectiveness for appetite suppression in its folklore use, together with research in animals and humans that demonstrate biologically active effects of some components of Hoodia on feeding behavior. This book would be incomplete without addressing some of the popular dietary supplements that may assist in weight control.

Hydroxycitric acid has been proposed as a natural substance that will inhibit fat storage, suppress appetite and decrease body weight.

The evidence for these effects is questionable. It has been suggested in a naïve manner that hydroxycitric acid may divert carbohydrates taken in the diet, away from their accumulation as body fat and promote their storage as glycogen. Glycogen stores are limited, and this explanation of the potential benefits of hydroxycitric acid is equally limited.

Much has been made of the use of derivatives of fatty acids such as conjugated linoleic acid (CLA) for weight control. While some laboratory evidence shows that CLA can enhance the mobilization of fatty acids, evidence for its actions alone in reducing weight is quite limited. Furthermore, rapid "mobilization" of fatty acids may be risky in some people.

Some companies have proposed the use of herbs or botanicals that may have some benefit in the control of blood glucose. For example, extracts of Lagerstroemia speciosa may stimulate glucose transport and assist in balancing blood sugar. This product may be useful in the metabolic Syndrome X and or the complementary management of Type 2 diabetes mellitus, but its role as weight loss supplement has little scientific support. Similar arguments apply to extracts of Coleus forskolii which is primarily used to support healthy blood sugar levels.

The proposal that L-carnitine can transport fats into mitochondria, where such fats could be consumed, is lacking in consistent scientific merit. The administration of chitosan as a fat blocker or cholesterol-lowering agent does not have strong support for a benefit in the scientific literature. The idea of blocking sugar absorption with so-called "starch blockers" is not a new concept, but the adjunctive use of extracts from the Phaseolus vulgaris bean may block sugar absorption by interfering with enzymes that break down starch in the small intestine. I believe that small amounts of starch blockers are valuable in giving an edge on simple sugar exclusion from the body, but they are not stand-alone weight loss agents. However, they may be useful in nutritional factors to combat Syndrome X and weight gain (www.naturesbenefit.com).

Among the many proposed alternatives to ephedra for use in dietary supplements, the stimulatory effects of green tea for weight control appear to be quite attractive and safe. Several studies have implied that extracts of green tea may be valuable in weight control by unknown mechanisms. Certainly, green tea contains caffeine, but there are other actions of green tea constituents that may benefit body metabolism and help to control weight (green tea polyphenols). Green tea may have beneficial effects on glucose metabolism.

Much of the evidence for the beneficial affects of green tea on health are derived from the use of green tea beverages in a traditional setting in Asian countries (www.greenteamax.com). Therefore, green tea leaves or extracts placed in capsules cannot be assumed to have the benefits of green tea when used as a standard beverage. There is no precedent of benefit for the combination of green tea leaves with Hoodia, but green tea polyphenol extracts could complement the actions of Hoodia gordonii on healthy weight control.

Green tea is not appealing to the Western palate, but several blends of green tea or liquid extracts of green tea with a pleasing flavor have become available for general use (www.greenteamax.com). These concentrates have a variable addition of other valuable antioxidants that may be beneficial in the management of the metabolic Syndrome X. I have used organic green tea concentrates combined with multiple antioxidants with significant reported benefits by individuals involved in aerobic exercise and healthy weight control tactics. The combination of organic, liquid green tea extracts has included the addition of turmeric, red clover, grape seed extract, pinebark extract, ellagic acid, citrus bioflavonoids, resveratrol, and selected oligomeric proanthocyanidins (www.greenteamax.com). Herbal teas have been used for years as dietary aids for weight control and green tea may be an ideal adjunct for weight loss in some individuals (www.greenteamax.com).

False Weight Loss Claims

False or misleading claims on weight loss products have been a specific focus of interest by regulatory agencies, such as the Food and Drug Administration (FDA) and the Federal Trade Commission (FTC) of the U.S. Over the past couple of years, the FDA and FTC have sent hundreds of warning letters to the marketers of weight loss products, especially those who primarily operate via the Internet. While there is no attractive single drug for the management of weight control, it is fair to say that there has been no single dietary supplement ingredient that can fulfill a promise of consistent healthy weight control. It remains to be seen whether or not Hoodia gordonii will fulfill its promise as a successful dietary supplement for general, healthy, and effective weight control.

Caveat Emptor: Emerging Hoodia Scams

At the time of writing, the interest in Hoodia gordonii, as a dietary supplement, has already swept the nation. Predictably, many dietary supplement companies are producing different brands of products that allegedly contain Hoodia gordonii from South Africa. These supplements carry a variable promise of biological activity. Internet advertising has become frenetic, deceptive in some circumstances, and positively corrupt in others. Many web pages contain false claims or misleading information about Hoodia, and its "form" in dietary supplements.

Some purveyors of dietary supplements are reckless enough to make frank "drug claims" or "hyperbolic statements". Readers should be aware that there is a great need to exercise discretion on the Hoodia they purchase. A dietary supplement containing Hoodia that contains plant material which is consistent in origin, pure, and of high quality is Hoodia Supreme™ (www.hoodiasupreme.com).

When any category of dietary supplement becomes very popular, there seems to be a small segment of the dietary supplement industry that disregards quality, purity and cost advantage of bulk reagents that are used to make a product. Quality dietary supplements containing Hoodia differ in this regard, because they contain material that is grown under strict quality control in an approved manner by cultivators who are supervised by the South African government (www.hoodiasupreme.com).

Is Hoodia gordonii an Endangered Plant?

In December 2004, directives about Hoodia came from South African government, supported by other responsible "bodies of opinion". These directives cautioned about the potential endangerment of the plant Hoodia gordonii, especially as commercial needs for this plant start to outstrip its availability. While Hoodia gordonii is not classified as an endangered plant, the response of the South African government has been to limit permission to export Hoodia gordonii from South Africa to certain companies.

Upon information and belief, there are only a few principle companies (at the time of writing) with South African Government Approved Permits to export Hoodia from South Africa. Only dietary supplements that have a consistent South African source of their active constituents should be used. These circumstances reinforce a strong need for purchasers of Hoodia gordonii to be aware of inferior and even fake products that may enter the dietary supplement markets (**caveat emptor**).

Many companies who intend to market Hoodia gordonii do not have a clear supply arrangement in place and it is unlikely that they will be able to produce in conformity any significant amount of a dietary supplement containing high quality Hoodia. Already, "cactus-like material" from Mexico, Arizona, and China has appeared as a bulk reagent that may be used in inferior — or fake — dietary supplements, labeled as Hoodia.

Safety of Hoodia Supplements

On the one hand no significant adverse effects of Hoodia have been reported, but on the other one cannot provide a "complete" safety seal for this dietary supplement or any other botanical supplement. Hoodia has been a "food" for centuries in South Africa, without reports of problems and with expressions of confidence in its nutritional value from native South African people. The precedent for the safety of Hoodia in adults is quite strong.

Dietary supplements containing Hoodia gordonii cannot be considered safe for use in childhood, pregnancy, or in lactating females who are breast feeding. It is not known if components of Hoodia enter breast milk and appetite suppression or other effects of Hoodia must be considered very undesirable in infants.

A great concern exists with Hoodia if it is abused or used by individuals with eating disorders that promote weight loss. Individuals with distorted body images who want to induce extreme degrees of weight loss often have a disorder called anorexia nervosa, with or without bulimia. Anorexia nervosa is becoming more common and it is a life-threatening disorder. Some comments have already been made in the media about the dangers of Hoodia use in the extreme "dieter" with an eating disorder.

A proposed "warning" for use with Hoodia gordonii as a dietary supplement would be "*Not to be used in childhood, pregnancy or lactating females who are breast feeding. Not to be used by individuals with eating disorders or those who are underweight or within a normal weight range. Allergic reactions may occur, as with all plant material. Reduced calorie intake can affect the control of diabetes mellitus. In cases of doubt, check with a medical practitioner prior to use.*"

Chapter Summary

The commercialization of Hoodia gordonii as a dietary supplement has created major interest. Hoodia should not be seen as some kind of "magic bullet for weight control".

Hoodia supplements present whole plants in a powdered form, most often in capsules or tablets. Using Hoodia in this manner is close to the original folklore use of Hoodia by the San bushmen in South Africa.

It has been proposed that the active components of Hoodia that suppress appetite are steroidal glycosides, but other constituents of Hoodia may contribute to its biological effects, or Hoodia may act on the body by mechanisms, other than those already proposed in scientific literature. Individuals who wish to use Hoodia as a dietary supplement should be vigilant about the source, quality and purity of the bulk reagents used to make dietary supplements (www.hoodiasupreme.com)

CHAPTER 9

HOODIA
FREQUENTLY ASKED QUESTIONS

Hoodia at a Glance

This chapter asks and answers questions about Hoodia gordonii. It provides a quick reference to the main facts about the use of Hoodia as a dietary supplement. It should be remembered that many "scientific questions" about Hoodia gordonii remain unanswered.

At the time of writing, thousands of people have reported successful appetite suppression, behavior modification and weight control with Hoodia in dietary supplements, but the consistency of its benefits have not been formally measured in this context. Anecdotal benefits of the use of Hoodia as a supplement cannot be taken as conclusive evidence of consistent benefit. That said, I believe that the described benefits of Hoodia as a dietary supplement have not occurred by chance alone.

The following sections in this chapter are frequently asked questions about Hoodia gordonii with answers that reflect what I believe to be credible sources of information. Not all information on Hoodia gordonii as a supplement can be considered credible; and I warn about some "drivel" on the internet. Some answers to questions about Hoodia involve a certain degree of speculation, on my part.

Question: What is Hoodia gordonii?
Answer: Hoodia gordonii is a cactus-like plant belonging to a group of plants that are described as succulents. Hoodia belongs to a botanical family of plants called Asclepiadaceae. Hoodia grows in the Kalahari desert of South Africa. This plant has been used for thousands of years by the San bushmen of South Africa to control hunger and thirst during hunting expeditions in the Kalahari desert.

Question: Who are the San bushmen?

Answer: The San people are the aboriginal people of Southern Africa. Their distinct hunter-gatherer culture stretches back over 20,000 years, and their genetic origins reach back over one million years. Recent research indicates that the San are the oldest genetic stock of contemporary humanity. Ten thousand years ago their exclusive domain stretched from the Zambezi to the Cape of Good Hope, from the Atlantic to the Indian Oceans. Three hundred years ago European colonists called them "untamable". Now Southern Africa's 110,000 remaining San face cultural extinction, living lives of poverty on the outer edges of society. Today they struggle to win back a foothold, along with their pride, in the lands they once roamed freely.

Question: What does Hoodia gordonii do?

Answer: Hoodia gordonii is presented as a powerful nutrional supplement for suppressing appetite, to be used with a calorie controlled diet and a healthy lifestyle, for healthy weight loss in individuals who are obese or overweight. This impressive plant contains special substances which act on the brain by sending a signal to tell the body that it is satisfied and does not need more food. Suggested usage for Hoodia is somewhat dependent upon body mass. A recommended dosage of 50-400 mg of pure Hoodia gordonii or a concentrate, one hour before meal times is a good general guideline. There are no reported side effects from the usage of Hoodia, other than lack of hunger and weight loss.

Question: How does Hoodia work in the body?

Answer: The Hoodia gordonii succulent plant has been used for centuries by the Xhomani San bushmen of Southern Africa's Kalahari desert, to suppress the appetite during long hunting trips. It works by making patients feel full after ingesting it, and it has been shown to lower food intake by up to 50% in small studies by pharmaceutical companies wishing to create a synthetic derivative from Hoodia (a drug). Although western scientists became aware of the plants potential about 75 years ago, it was only recently that the putative active ingredients of Hoodia have been patented by the South African Council for Scientific and Industrial Research.

Subsequently, a British biotechnology company, Phytopharm acquired the rights to the further development and commercialization of Hoodia components as an anti-obesity drug for use in the West. Now the San people, in the first deal of its kind, will be rewarded for the development of a drug which makes use of their traditional knowledge. Under the terms of the agreement, the San people will receive regular fees as the drug developed from a plant, used to suppress the appetite, passes various stages on the way to market.

Question: How did Hoodia become so popular so quickly?

Answer: The media has covered the startling effects of Hoodia on appetite and weight control over the past 18 months. Ranging from newspaper articles to TV shows, the interest in Hoodia has swept the US nation and countries in Western Europe. In one interview reported by ABC news, a spokesman for the San people who live in the Kalahari desert, Andries Steenkamp says, " *I learned how to eat it from my fore-fathers,*" as he prepared a piece of the cactus-like plant called Hoodia by trimming off the prickly spikes. *" It is my food, my water, and also a medicine for me".* *"Hoodia stops hunger and also treats sickness"* Steenkamp told ABC news. *"We San, use the plant during hunting to fight off the pain of hunger and thirst."* There are no known side effects with Hoodia gordonii although it is said to possess a mild aphrodisiac effect. It contains no ephedra or caffeine or any other stimulants.

Other TV broadcasts on the shows "60 minutes" and "20/20" have fueled the popularity of Hoodia gordonii in early 2005. The first TV reporters' experiences were recorded by the BBC. A BBC correspondent, Tom Mangold, described "the cactus test". The following is an abstract of Tom Mangold's report. *"In order to see for ourselves, we drove into the desert, four hours north of Cape town in search of the cactus. Once there, we found an unattractive plant which sprouts about 10 tentacles, and is the size of a long cucumber. Each tentacle is covered in spikes which needs to be carefully peeled. Inside is a slightly unpleasant-tasting, fleshy plant. At about 18 00 hours, I ate about half a banana size-piece and later so did my cameraman. Soon after, we began the four hour drive back to Cape town. The plant is said to have a feel-good almost aphrodisiac quality, and I have to say, we felt good. But more significantly, we did not even think about food. Our brains really were telling us we were full. It was a magnificent deception. Dinner time came and went. We reached our hotel at about midnight and went to bed without food. And the next day, neither of us wanted, nor ate breakfast. I ate lunch but without appetite and very little pleasure. Partial, then full appetite returned slowly after 24 hours.*"

Question: Are all Hoodia supplements of the same quality?

Answer: Hoodia plants are native to the semi-arid deserts of South Africa, Botswana, Namibia and Angola. Even though there are about 20 species in the Hoodia family, the gordonii species may be the principal one that contains natural appetite suppressants. This means that only Hoodia from South Africa can be expected to have potential appetite suppressant and weight control benefits. Dietary supplements containing cactus-like material from China or Mexico or the U.S. must be considered "fakes". This "fake" material is being used in some dietary supplements sold, as "Hoodia," upon information and belief.

Question: Is there scientific support for Hoodia's effects on weight control?

Answer: When South African scientists were testing the Hoodia plant, they discovered the plant contained previously unknown molecules that cause a sensation of "fullness" (satiety). Results of human clinical trials in Britain suggest that this active ingredient could reduce the appetite and reduce dietary intake of calories by up to one to two thousand calories a day. Active ingredients in Hoodia work by replicating the effect glucose has on nerve cells in the brain (hypothalamus), fooling the body into thinking it is full, even when it is not. Hoodia appears to contain a molecule that is almost 10,000 times stronger than glucose, in its effects on brain to cause a feeling of "fullness "(satiety).

Early animal experiments in free-feeding rats have shown that the administration of Hoodia gordonii reduced the amount that they ate. Rats are greedy, with a voracious appetite, and they will eat almost anything. Altering the feeding habits of rats with Hoodia was a striking experimental finding. Reductions in food intakes in rats have been demonstrated repeatedly in experiments performed in South Africa, England and the United States.

Following the rat experiments, human clinical trials were performed in an obese group of people who were placed in a strictly enforced environment. These overweight people were left to eat as much as they liked, watch television, and read. Half of this group of obese individuals was given Hoodia gordonii and half were given a placebo (dummy pill). Fifteen days later, the group of subjects receiving Hoodia had significantly reduced their calorie intake. These experiments were a stunning success, because weight loss accompanied the loss of appetite and reduction of dietary calorie intake in these people.

Question: What is the reaction of the San people to the commercialization of Hoodia?

Answer: The San bushmen believe strongly that the effect of Hoodia on appetite is their discovery but they had to fight big business interests to be included in revenue sharing from the commercial success of Hoodia. The San people are now working with cultivators in South Africa and they are benefiting with jobs, given the popularity of this plant. *"The San people, in the first deal of its kind, will be rewarded for the development of a drug which makes use of their traditional knowledge. Under the terms of this agreement, the San people will receive regular fees as the drug developed from a plant used to suppress the appetite passes various stages on the way to market. The San people hailed the agreement as a joyous moment. Mr Chennells, lawyer for the San people in negotiating the export of the Hoodia gordonii plant is ecstatic: The San will finally throw off thousands of years of oppression, poverty, social isolation and discrimination. We will create a trust fund with their Hoodia royalties and the children will join South Africa's middle classes in our lifetime."*

Question: Are extracts of Hoodia used in dietary supplements?

Answer: No. At the time of writing, some dietary supplements have been mislabeled as containing extracts. There is some form of concentration used in processing the whole Hoodia plant in some cases, but standardized extracts are not readily available. The extraction process to obtain active steroidal glycoside molecules from Hoodia gordonii is a patented process, used only by scientists involved in drug development programs. Products that are labeled "pure Hoodia gordonii" are to be preferred. In simple terms, there is no such thing such as standardized extract of Hoodia in the dietary supplement industry and the preparation and sale of such extracts would be illegal and a clear breach of patents held by business corporations, including but not limited to Phytopharm PLC of England. The food giant Unilever Inc. has stated that it has patent rights to use extracts in food products, after further research and development.

Question: How would one select the best Hoodia supplement?

Answer: Purchase Hoodia only from a company that will guarantee that the source of the whole plant is South Africa. Use Hoodia supplements that contain at least 200mg of Hoodia gordonii powder. Superior Hoodia supplements usually contain at least 400mg of whole Hoodia powder, preferably in vegetable capsules (www.hoodia-supreme.com). Bulk suppliers of whole Hoodia plants are not routinely testing for steroidal glycoside content. Selling a Hoodia supplement on the basis of its steroidal glycoside content would be considered patent infringement. The reality is that dietary supplements containing whole Hoodia powder are sold on the understanding that the whole plant is used in a somewhat similar manner to the way in which the San bushmen took the plant in their diet.

Question: Is Hoodia gordonii an endangered plant?

Answer: At the time of writing, there was some evidence that the demand for Hoodia had outstripped its supply. There are conventions governing international trade in any species of wild plants. Hoodia gordonii cultivation and export is being carefully regulated by the South African government and Hoodia has been listed in documents that form international agreements between governments to make sure that international trade in certain plants will not threaten their survival, overall. Companies importing Hoodia to the United States from South Africa must import Hoodia material with a South African government approved export permit.

Question: Will the supply of Hoodia for dietary supplements be sustainable?

Answer: Export permits must be purchased for all material containing Hoodia gordonii that leaves Africa. The South African government is now strictly controlling these permits. The money from the sale of these permits supports economic development initiatives for African tribes, including the San bushmen. Responsible suppliers of Hoodia in South Africa are in the process of negotiating transactions with the South African San Institute to develop nurseries that are operated by San bushmen and their families. These nurseries are being developed to supply seedlings that can be used to stock outlying farming projects.

Legal considerations have led growers and their brokers to avoid much reference to the San bushmen in their commercial activity. There has been a preference to speak in terms of financial contributions to economic development projects for South African people, rather than to talk specifically about the San bushmen.

Question: Is there official evidence of the sustainability of Hoodia supply?

Answer: There are companies involved in cultivation of Hoodia gordonii, but there may only be a small number of these operations that carry legitimate permits to cultivate and harvest Hoodia gordonii. Responsible growers of Hoodia are investing in land and already planting new Hoodia seedlings. It is reported that for the remainder of the year 2005, the only supply of Hoodia supreme will come from commercially propagated crops of Hoodia. It is stated among horticulturists that Hoodia needs about three years to mature, to be reliable in terms of its content of biologically active material.

Question: Are tests conducted on Hoodia raw material used in dietary supplements?

Answer: In brief, some material is tested, but most is not, upon information and belief. Hoodia gordonii supplied by agricultural operations in South Africa, that employ experts in "succulent horticulture" try to ensure that their stock of seedling is gathered from authentic sources in the Kalahari desert. These experts are charged with the responsibility of verifying that the Hoodia grown is of the gordonii variety. Therefore, material imported from Mexico or China cannot be taken seriously, as a source of bioactive Hoodia.

Responsible suppliers test material using an independent laboratory, and verify that the raw material contains the necessary components for the actions of Hoodia. These factors have been very important in deciding on the type of bulk material that I recommend for inclusion in dietary supplements. Pure Hoodia is used as a source of material found in the product Hoodia Supreme™ (www.hoodiasupreme.com).

Question: Is Hoodia gordonii patented?

Answer: The "plant" Hoodia gordonii cannot be patented for any reason, in itself, or in its whole form. It has been known for many years that

Hoodia gordonii has appetite and thirst -suppressing properties, as well as energizing and possible aphrodisiac effects. What is clearly patented are putative active constituents of Hoodia gordonii and related compounds that belong to a group of chemicals called steroidal glycosides. Dietary supplements should not be sold with claims about steroidal glycoside content, per se. Growers of Hoodia gordonii in South Africa and the San bushmen have argued that "the whole plant" has not been patented. One major supplier of Hoodia reports that Hoodia gordonii is classified as a "natural food product" by the South African government.

In the U.S., dietary supplements are not food and they are not considered to be drugs. Dietary supplements are permitted to be used if there was evidence of their use in the food chain prior to 1994 when the Dietary Supplement and Health Education Act was placed into legislation. There is no doubt that Hoodia gordonii was used in the South African food chain prior to 1994, but some have questioned whether or not Hoodia was used as a food prior to 1994, in the U.S.

It is difficult to pinpoint evidence of the use of Hoodia prior to 1994 in the U.S., but there may evidence that cactus-like or succulent plant material has been eaten in the United States for many years. Indeed, other types of cactus have found their way into dietary supplements in the United States.

The main issue is whether or not Hoodia gordonii is considered to be safe. The longstanding use of Hoodia in the food chain of South African native people, over as long as several centuries or more, seems to be a powerful precedent for the safety of Hoodia gordonii and some related species of Hoodia.

Question: Is Hoodia for everyone?

Answer: Absolutely not. Hoodia gordonii is best used in mature adults. It should be avoided in childhood, pregnancy and when a lactating female is breastfeeding. When anyone takes herbs or botanical supplements, there is always a risk of an allergic reaction, but I can find no reports of allergic reactions to Hoodia gordonii. However, the chances are that occasional people may have or develop an allergy.

Although Hoodia has been described as a "miracle", containing "miracle molecules", it cannot be seen as a "magic bullet" for the global epidemic of obesity or overweight problems. The value of Hoodia appears to be its ability to suppress appetite in an almost "passive manner". With the failure of many fad diets and many drugs or dietary supplements for weight control, scientists and the general public are realizing that weight loss efforts must go "back to basics". The key issue in weight control is reduction of calorie intake, and this is what happens in many people when Hoodia is taken as a dietary supplement, or in medical research, where extracts of Hoodia gordonii have been given to both animals and humans in drug development experiments, with beneficial weight loss results.

Question: How did, or do, the San really use Hoodia gordonii?
Answer: The San bushmen find the idea of the use of Hoodia for weight loss to be a contrarian thought. The San bushmen were traditionally lean and supremely fit individuals who used Hoodia only to endure their terrible ordeal of desperate requirements for food. More recently, it is reported that San bushmen have embraced western lifestyle and indeed there are a number of native people in South Africa who have problems with obesity and the metabolic Syndrome X. It is reported that the San have been using Hoodia recently to overcome obesity problems, especially in their children. This is a major shift in the ethno-botanical use of Hoodia gordonii.

Question: What are the key commercial questions about Hoodia gordonii?
Answer: Much discussion is occurring about the sustainability of supply of Hoodia gordonii, its quality control during growth and processing, its evidence of effectiveness, questions on how it should be regulated?, and what is its overall safety?. One must speculate in some areas of these important questions. The quality of bulk Hoodia material used in dietary supplements has emerged as extremely variable and some evidence exists that fake, cactus-like material may be used by some marketing predators who want to "cash in" on the "Hoodia bandwagon".

The effectiveness of Hoodia supplements in assisting with weight control requires more research, before firm conclusions can be drawn. That said, there are many testimonials of effective weight control with the use of Hoodia. Many of these testimonials have involved the person in question complying with a calorie controlled diet and healthy lifestyle change. Much information is required from future research of Hoodia gordonii.

Question: Will Hoodia affect blood insulin or blood glucose levels?

Answer: The mechanism of action of Hoodia on the brain may work through receptors in the hypothalamus of the brain that respond to prevailing blood glucose concentrations in the body. However, I, and others have described other potential mechanisms of action of Hoodia, in addition to its effect on glucose sensing by the brain. The constituents of Hoodia gordonii do not seem to affect prevailing blood insulin concentrations by direct mechanisms, but changes in blood glucose and insulin levels can be expected when a calorie-reduced diet reduces sugar intake which, in turn, will reduce prevailing blood glucose concentrations and blood insulin levels. Therefore, the effects of Hoodia on blood glucose or blood insulin are most likely to be indirect effects.

I proposed a unique combination of Hoodia gordonii with coffee bean extract, containing chlorogenic acid in this book. Again, there will be at least an indirect effect on blood glucose and insulin levels with this combination, as described in Chapter 7.

Question: Does Hoodia gordonii interact with medications?

Answer: There is not much information available on this subject and I can find no specific descriptions of drug interactions with Hoodia gordonii, at the time of writing. However, any reduction in calorie consumption or food intake may be expected to alter the control of obesity-related diseases such as diabetes mellitus. Therefore, weight loss must be considered as altering the clinical course or natural history of some diseases. In brief, weight loss in the obese individual has many more advantages than disadvantages and this is the overall goal in the combat against weight gain.

Summarizing Hoodia and its Use in South Africa

Hoodia plants look like large cucumbers with protruding, small thorns along their stems. These Hoodia plants are leafless and the stems of the plants contain fleshy material with high water content. Hoodia plants have pinkish or flesh-colored flowers that look like small TV reception dishes. I have referred to Hoodia plants as "stinky". They have an odor similar to rotten meat or a "food garbage" smell. This unpleasant odor attracts flies and blowflies, which lay eggs inside the "rotten-smelling" flowers of the plant. This process of egg-laying by insects results in pollination of the succulent plants.

There are many varieties of plants in South Africa that are pollinated in this unique manner by insects. Understanding pollination of the succulents has led to the use of botanical terms to describe flowering portions of these plants as "carrion-flowers", or "stapeliads". I mention these detailed botanical facts to point out that it is difficult to identify different species of Hoodia, without considerable knowledge of the structure of these plants. The variability of appearance of succulent plants, with some degree of common architectural features, results in difficulty of identification of the correct Hoodia species that should be harvested to make supplements containing Hoodia gordonii or other active Hoodia species.

Species of Hoodia within the overall family of plants called Asclepiadaceae include: Hoodia currorii, otherwise known by the confusing names *GHAAP, !Khobab, and Khoi,* Hoodia gordonii or *bitterghaap,* Hoodia fluva, or *yellow-flowered ghaap,* Hoodia officinalis, Hoodia lugardii, and Hoodia pilifera. These latter types of Hoodia have been generally referred to as *ghaap* and all types of Hoodia are sometimes called *"South African desert cactus",* even though these plants are not examples of a true cactus.

There has been much confusion among South African farmers, and people who have used Hoodia as food, when it comes to the specific recognition of the species of Hoodia that is being used in their diet. It is recorded that two principle types of *ghaap* were first recognized by botanists. The first was called *"true ghaap",* which is a group of plants believed to be part of a genus of plants called Trichocaulon of different species. The second has been referred to as *bobbejaanghaap,* and this unusual name is often applied to Hoodia species in general. Scientists have made remarks about the considerable overlap between these two groups of plants, and this has resulted in uniting Trichocaulon species and Hoodia species under the single genus of Hoodia. This unification of different types of succulents was proposed in 1993 (Bruyns, 1993), according to South African, botanical records.

Circumstances become even more confusing when other plants are called *"ghaap".* It has been noted that other succulent plants, or plants with carrion-flowers (stapeliads), are sometimes called *"ghaap"* or have names that are interchangeable with names given to species of Hoodia. For example, a plant called "Pectinaria maurghamii" is sometimes referred to as "*ghaap*" by local people. While all of these names are confusing, I reiterate the difficulty that there may be in identifying different species of Hoodia plants.

It is clear that Hoodia species have been eaten by many South African citizens, other than the aboriginal San bushmen. Farmers in the Northern Cape of South Africa have used Hoodia species as a backup source of food and water at times of food emergencies. There is a tradition for shepherds on farms to eat Hoodia for its appetite and thirst-suppressing qualities, but this use of Hoodia was originated by the San bushmen, according to history and folklore.

South African people who eat Hoodia, prefer to eat the stems of this plant after episodes of significant rainfall. At these times, the Hoodia plant is swollen and contains much water. The plant is eaten by scraping the spines off the stems of plants, with a knife or stone. Local people may pick Hoodia and soak it in water before it is eaten. This may dull some of the bitter taste of Hoodia, and ensure that the water-retaining fiber or mucilage components of the stem are fully hydrated.

In this book, I have focused on the reported appetite-suppressing effects of Hoodia, but South African native people have used Hoodia to treat indigestion, manage diabetes mellitus, reduce blood pressure, and manage stomach-aches. Some species of Hoodia produce an aftertaste in the mouth, rather like the flavor of anis or licorice. It is reported that this aftertaste produced by Hoodia gives tobacco smoke a very pleasant taste and sensation. Hoodia should not be used to promote smoking addictions that damage health.

It is interesting to speculate what may be "real" in terms of the health benefits of Hoodia species. Certainly, the use of Hoodia for indigestion seems to be supported by the knowledge that certain molecules, found in Hoodia species, may inhibit acid secretion by the stomach (Chapter 8). There are reports that Hoodia gordonii has been taken as a "traditional medicine" for abdominal pain of the variety that may occur in association with peptic ulceration of the upper digestive tract.

Whether or not Hoodia lowers blood pressure remains to be defined. One could anticipate favorable effects of Hoodia on Type II diabetes mellitus, if calorie control occurs in the diet, together with sugar restriction, as a result of the appetite-suppressing effects of Hoodia. There is some suggestion that Hoodia gordonii can have paradoxical effects on appetite, where appetite stimulation has been described in some circumstances of severe hunger? Finally, a specific species of Hoodia (notably, Hoodia officinalis) has been used to treat pulmonary tuberculosis, and even hemorrhoids.

The value of Hoodia in the management of pulmonary tuberculosis is not clear, but the use of Hoodia as a remedy for hemorrhoids was documented to have occurred in the United States prior to 1994. How Hoodia was administered or taken for hemorrhoid management in the U.S. is not clear, but this provides evidence that Hoodia species may have been used in the "food or supplement chain" prior to the "magic date" of 1994, when the assent of the Dietary Supplement and Health Education Act occurred (DSHEA, 1994). This information was documented by Bruyns in 1993; and it may form a clear basis to accept Hoodia species from South Africa as "grandfathered" as a dietary supplement. In addition, Hoodia pilifera was reported to suppress hunger and thirst in the 1960's (Smith, 1966). It is noted that stems of the succulent plant Hoodia pilifera were mixed with alcohol to create tinctures that were used to treat indigestion, stomach-ache, hemorrhoids, and even pulmonary tuberculosis.

Hoodia species are well accepted as "traditional medicines" in South Africa and they carry the label of "health food" or "functional food". It has to be recognized that the characterization of Hoodia species and their biological effects remains a matter of incomplete understanding, but Hoodia seems to qualify as a very useful dietary supplement.

Chapter Summary

This chapter poses questions on Hoodia gordonii and attempts to answer them. These frequently asked questions and their answers should permit readers to obtain a rapid overview of the characteristics and potential use of Hoodia gordonii as a dietary supplement. Some of the material presented in this chapter was provided by D. Vickary of Stella Labs Inc., NJ and used with permission. The consumer writings of D. Vickary are gratefully acknowledged.

AFTERWORD

Medical practitioners and obese individuals are becoming increasingly disenchanted with promises of new diets, new drugs, and new dietary supplements for weight control. The American public must now be tired of being told that they are overweight, obese, and unfit. Weight control is now a very serious business, as there is increasing recognition that weight gain poses a major threat to the health and well-being of modern humankind. Obesity is accompanied by many "ugly" disease companions. One could fill a page of text with a list of the complications and disease associations of obesity. No longer can we think about our overweight status in a unitary manner.

The tragic epidemic of the metabolic Syndrome X is a terrifying threat to western society. About 70 million American people have the variable combination of excessive fat storage in the body, associated with high blood cholesterol, and high blood pressure. This constellation of problems is linked together in the metabolic syndrome by the frequent occurrence of resistance to the hormone insulin.

Just losing weight, just lowering blood pressure, just lowering blood cholesterol, or just treating glucose intolerance are not enough to reduce premature death and disability that is frequently encountered in the metabolic Syndrome X. Therefore, the overweight individual or obese person has more to think about than merely waistline reduction. Weight loss is no longer a primary, cosmetic issue. Obesity is a major challenge to health, and this disease "hangs out" with many health challenging problems.

No wonder many overweight people have become desperate when they respond to the promises of a new, effective, weight control strategy that does not deliver the required outcome. The majority of people who adopt any weight control diet will regain weight, often within a year after the initiation of the diet. Diets are not stand-alone interventions for weight control, and equally, drugs or dietary supplements are not consistently effective when used alone to fight the flab. Effective weight control has to have a primary initiative of health, not just weight loss. Weight control is a function of healthy lifestyle, calorie controlled diets, with the selection of healthy foods, and expenditure of energy by the body, with appropriate levels of exercise. Behavior modification is a key issue for sustained weight control. The examination of groups of individuals who have successfully controlled their weight over extended periods of time reveals that these individuals have taken a multi-pronged approach to weight management.

A pivotal issue in weight control is looking at the amount of energy taken into the body in the form of food. A significant proportion of the U.S. nation has engaged in wishful thinking when they accept the nonsensical statement that: *"calories do not count."* A calorie is a form of energy derived from food that can be stored by the body as fat. The promise of Hoodia is great, when scientists observe that the administration of Hoodia gordonii, or selected extracts of this plant, result in significant reductions of calorie intake in both animals and humans in a manner that can be replicated in scientific experiments. Hoodia gordonii heralds a new weight loss revolution where weight control must go "back to basics" with resolution and commitment for weight control in the obese individual. Many people are hoping that Hoodia gordonii will live up to its promise of being a "miracle of nature" to help us manage our recalcitrant weight gain.

REFERENCES (Principle references only listed):

Anand BK, Brobeck JR (1951) *Hypothalamic control of food intake in rats and cats.* Yale J. Bio. Med. 24:123-133.

Anderson GH (1979) *Control of protein and energy intake: role of plasma amino acids and neurotransmitters.* Can. J. Physiol. Phamacol. 57:1043-1057.

Anderson GH (1994) *Regulation of food intake.* In Shils ME, Olson JA, Shike M (eds), *Modern nutrition in health and disease,* 8th ed. Lea & Febiger, Malvern, pp 524-536.

Anderson GH (1995) *Sugars, sweetness, and food intake.* Am. J. Clin. Nutr. 62(suppl): 195S-202S.

Anderson GH, Black RM, Li ETS (1992) *Physiologic determinants of food selection: association with protein and carbohydrate.* In Anderson GH, Kennedy SH (eds), *The biology of feast and famine: relevance to eating disorders.* Academic Press, Toronto, pp 73-91.

Anderson GH, Li ETS, Glanville NT (1984) *Brain mechanisms and the quantitative and qualitative aspects of food intake.* Brain Res. Bull. 12:167-173.

Angel, R.L. Hauger, MD Luu, B Giblin, P Skolnick, SM Paul, *Glucostatic regulation of (+)-[3H]amphetamine binding in the hypothalamus: correlation with Na+, K+-ATPase activity,* Proc. Natl. Acad. Sci. U. S. A. 82 (1985) 6320-6324.

Black R, Anderson GH (1994) *Sweeteners, food intake and selection.* In Fernstrom JD, Miller G (eds), *Appetite and body weight regulation: sugar, fat and macronutrient substitutes.* CRC Press, Boca Raton, pp 125-136.

Blundell JE, Green S, Burley V (1994) *carbohydrates and human appetite.* Am. J. Clin. Nutr. 59(suppl):728S-734S.

Booth DA (1972) *Conditioned satiety in the rat.* J Comp Physiol Psych 81:457-471.

Campfield LA, Smith FJ, 1990 *Transient declines in blood glucose signal meal initiation.* Int J Obes 14 suppl 3:15-33

Castonguay TW, Stern JS (1990) *Hunger and appetite.* In Brown M (ed), *Present knowledge in nutrition,* 6th ed. International Life Sciences Institute, Washington, DC, pp13-22.

Dam R M and Feskens E J M, *Coffee consumption and risk of type Z diabetes mellitus* Lancet, 2002.

Drewnowski A (1994) *Human preferences for sugar and fat.* In Fernstorm JD, Miller GD (eds), *Appetite and body weight regulation.* CRC Press, Boca Raton, pp 137-147.

Flatt J-P (1993) *Dietary fat, carbohydrate balance and weight maintenance.* Ann N Y Acad Sci 683:122-140.

Flatt J-P (1995) *Use and storage of fat and carbohydrate.* Am. J. Clin. Nutr. 61(suppl)952S-959S.

Ford ES, Giles WH and Dietz WH, *Prevalence of the Metabolic Syndrome (Syndrome X) Among US Adults*, JAMA 287, 3, 356-359, 2002. Mayer J, 1955 *Regulation of energy intake and the body weight, the glucostatis theory and the lipostatic hypothesis*, Ann NY Acad Sci 63:15-43

Friedman MI (1990) *Body fat and the metabolic control of food intake*. Int J Obes 14(suppl)3:53-67.

Friedman MI, Rawson NE 1994, *Fuel metabolism and appetite control. In Fernstrom JD, Miller GD eds, Appetite and body weight regulation: sugar, fat and macronutrient substitutes*. CRC Press, Boca Raton, pp 63-76.

Geitzen DW, 1993, *Neural mechanism in the responses to amino acid deficiency*. J Nutr 1223:610-625

Geliebter AA (1979) *Effects of equicaloric loads of protein, fat, and carbohydrate on food intake in the rat and man*. Physiol. Behav. 22:267-273.

Gerozissis M, Orosco M, Rouch C, et al, 1993, *Basal and hyperinuslinemia-induced immunoreactive hypothalamic insulin changes in lean and genetically obese Zucker rats revealed by microdialysis*. Brain Res 611:258-263

Gietzen DW, 1986 *Time course of food intake and plasma and brain amino acid concentrations in rats fed amino acid imbalanced or-deficient diets*. In Morley JE, Kave R, Brand JG eds, Interaction of the chemical sense with nutrition. Academic Press, New York, pp415-456,

Gupta, SP *Quantitative structure-activity relationships of cardiotonic agents*, Prog. Drug Res. 55 (2000) 235-282.

H. Ji, M.I. Friedman, *Compensatory hyperphagia after fasting tracks recovery of liver energy status*, Physiol. Behav. 68 (1999) 181-186.

Hakkin J, et al, US Patent No.: 6,488,967, inventors Hakkinen J, et al, assigned to Phytopharm PLC of Godmanchester, UK. This patent describes a method of treating disease or disorders of the gastrointestinal tract using extracts of plants of the genus Hoodia or Trichocaulon or related chemical compounds.

Hamilton BS, Paglia D, Kwan AYM, et al 1995, *Increased obese m-RNA expression in omental fat cells from massively obese humans*, Nature Med 1:953-956

Heller RF, Heller RF, 1994, *Hyperinsulinemic obesity and carbohydrate addiction: the missing link is the carbohydrate frequency factor*. Med Hypothese 42:307-312

Hill JO, Prentice AM (1995) *Sugar and body weight regulation* Am. J. Clin. Nutr. 62(suppl):264S-274S.

Horton ES (1983) *An overview of the assessment and regulation of energy balance in humans*. Am. J. Clin. Nutr. 38:972-977.

Horton TJ, Drougas H, Brachey A, et al (1995) *Fat and carbohydrate overfeeding in humans: different effects on energy storage*. Am Soc Clin Nutr 62:19-29.

Kalra, SP, Dube MG, Pu S, Xu B, Horvath TL, Kalra PS, *Interacting appetite-regulating pathways in the hypothalamic regulation of body weight*, Endoc. Rev. 20 (1999) 68-100.

Kren V, Martinkova L, *glycosides in medicine: The role of glycosidic residue in biological activity*, Curr. Med. Chem. 8 92001) 1303-1328.

Landsberg L (1994) *Pathophysiology of obesity-related hypertension: role of insulin and the sympathetic nervous system.* J. Cardiovasc. Pharmacol. 23(suppl)1:S1-S8.

Leibowitz SF (1994) *Specificity of hypothalamic peptides in the control of behavioral and physiological processes.* Ann N Y Acad Sci 739: 12-35.

Li ETS, Anderson GH (1982) *Meal composition influences subsequent food selection in the young rat.* Physiol. Behav. 29:779-783.

Lissner L, Heitmann BL (1995) *Dietary fat and obesity: evidence from epidemiology.* Eur J Clin Nutr 49:79-90.

Luo S, Trigazis L, Pang MB, et al (1994) *The effect of carbohydrate on short-term food intake in rats.* Int J Obes 18(suppl2):519.

Mayer J, 1980 *Physiology of hunger and satiety.* In Goodhart RS, Schils ME eds, *Modern nutrition and disease,* 6th ed. Lea & Febiger, Philadelphia, pp 560-577

McGee CD, Greenwood CE (1990) *Protein and carbohydrate selection respond to changes in dietary saturated fatty acids but not to changes in essential fatty acids.* Life Sci 47:67-76.

McGowan MK, Andrews KM, Grossman SB, 1992, *Chronicintrahy-pothalamic infusions of insulin or insulin antibodies alter body weight and food intake in rats.* Physiol Behave 51:753-756

McHugh PR, Moran TH (1985) *The stomach: a conception of its dynamic role in satiety.* Prog. Psychobiol. Physiol. Psychol. 11:197-232.

MacLean D, Lu-Guang L, *Increased ATP Content/production in the hypothalamus may be a signal for energy-sensing of society: studies of the anorectic mechanism of a plant steroidal glycoside,* Brain Research 1020 (2004) 1-11

Mellinkoff SM, Frankland M, Boyle D, et al, 1956 *Relationship between serum amino acid concentration and fluctuations in appetite.* J Appl Physiol 8:535-538

Mullen BJ, Martin RJ (1992) *The effect of dietary fat on diet selection may involve central serotonin.* Am J Physiol 263:R559-R563.

Nicoll RA, Alger B.E. *The Brian's Own Marijuana,* Scientific American, Dec. 2004, pp70-75

Raben. A, Christensen NJ, Madsen J, et al (1994) *Decreased postprandial thermogenesis and fat oxidation but increased fullness after a high-fiber meal compared with a low-fiber meal.* Am. J. Clin. Nutr. 59:1386-1394.

Read N, French S, Cunningham K (1994) *The role of the gut in regulating food intake in man.* Nutr Rev 52:1-10.

Rodriguez de Sotillo D.V., Hadley M, *Chlorogenic acid modifies plasma and liver concentrations of: cholesterol, triacylgycerol, and minerals in (fa/fa)Zucker rats,* Journal of Nutrional Biochemistry, 2002, Vol.13, No. 12, pp 717-726

Rolls BJ, Kim-Harris S, Fischman MW, et al (1994) *satiety after preloads with different amounts of fat and carbohydrate: implications for obesity.* Am J Clin Nutr 60:476-487.

Rozin P, Vollmecke TA (1986) *Food likes and dislikes.* Annu. Rev. Nutr. 6:433-456.

Schwartz MW, Figlewicz DP, Woods SC, et al 1993 *Insulin, neuropeptide Y, and food intake.* Ann NY Acad Sci 692:60-71

Strominger JL, Brobeck JR (1953) *A mechanism of regulation of food intake.* Yale J. Biol. Med. 25: 383-390.

Wogan GN, Marletta MA (1985) *Undesired or potentially undesirable constituents of foods.* In Fennema OR (ed), Food chemistry. Marcel Dekker, New York, pp 694-695.

Wurtman JJ, Moses PL, Wurtman RJ (1983) *Prior carbohydrate consumption affects the amount of carbohydrate that rats choose to eat.* J. Nutr. 113:70-78.

BOOKS BY THE AUTHOR

Skinner HA, Holt S, *The Alcohol Clinical Index*, Addiction Research Foundation, Toronto, 1993

Holt S, *Soya for Health*, Mary Ann Liebert Publishers, NY 1996

Holt S, and Comac L, *Miracle Herbs*, Carol Publishing, NJ 1997

Holt S and Barilla J, *The Power of Cartilage*, Kensington Publishers, NY 1998

Holt S, *The Sexual Revolution*, ProMotion Publishing, San Diego, California 1999

Holt S, *The Soy Revolution*, Dell Publishing, Random House, NY, NY, 1999 (third printing 2002)

Holt S, *Natural Ways to Digestive Health*, M. Evans Inc., NY, 2000 (second printing 2002)

Holt S, The Natural Way to a Healthy Heart, M. Evans and Co. Inc, NY, 1999 (second printing 2002)

Holt S and Bader D, *Natures Benefit for Pets*, Wellness Publishing, Newark NJ, 2001

Holt S, *Natures Benefit From Coral Calcium: Sorting Science from Speculation*, Wellness Publishing, Newark, NJ, 2002, First edition; 2003 Second edition

Holt S, *The Antiporosis Plan*, Wellness Publishing, Newark, NJ 2002

Holt S, *Combat Syndrome X, Y, and Z*, Wellness Publishing, Newark, NJ, 2002

Holt S, *Digestion*, Wellness Publishing, Newark NJ, 2005 (in press)

Holt S, Wright J, *Syndrome X Nutritional Factors*, Wellness Publishing, Newark NJ, 2004

Holt S, *The MenoPlan*, Wellness Publishing, Newark NJ, 2005 (in press)

Holt S, *Enhancing Low Carb Diets*, Wellness Publishing, Newark NJ, 2004

Holt S, *Sleep Naturally*, Wellness Publishing, Newark NJ, 2003

Dr. Holt's books are available in major bookstores, fine health food stores, and on the internet at www.wellnesspublishing.com